# "... AND YOU SHALL LIVE BY THEM"

## Contemporary Jewish Approaches to Medical Ethics

Louis Flancbaum, MD

MIRKOV PUBLICATIONS, INC.

Pittsburgh, Pennsylvania

MIRKOV PUBLICATIONS, INC.
P.O. Box 81971
Pittsburgh, Pennsylvania 15217
1-(800)-851-8303



Library of Congress Catalog Card Number 00-134269

10 9 8 7 6 5 4 3 2 1



ISBN 0-9648508-4-2

Manufactured in the United States of America

To My Beloved Parents

**Yetta and Max Flancbaum**

"What God is to the world, parents are to their children"

(Philo, *Honor Due to Parents*)

## TABLE OF CONTENTS

**Abbreviations**

ARR – American Reform Responsa (R. Walter Jacob)

Ar HaSh – *Aruch HaShulchan* (19th-century Code of Law by R. Y.M. Epstein)

BCE - Before Common Era (similar to BC)

BT - Babylonian Talmud

CARR – Contemporary American Reform Responsa (R. Walter Jacob)

CCAR – Central Conference of Reform Rabbis

CE - Common Era (similar to AD)

CJLS – Proceedings of the Committee on Jewish Law and Standards of the Conservative Movement

IM – *Iggrot Moshe* (Responsa of R. Moshe Feinstein, zt"l)

JT - Jerusalem Talmud

LA – *Lev Avraham* (medical ethics work by Dr. A.S. Abraham, containing many responsa of R. Shlomo Zalman Auerbach that were otherwise not published)

MB - *Mishnah B'rurah* (20th-century commentary on *Shulchan Aruch* by R. Israel Meir Kagan)

MRR – Modern Reform Responsa (R. Solomon B. Freehof)

MT - *Mishneh Torah* (Maimonides' Code of Jewish Law)

NA – *Nishmat Avraham* (medical ethics work by Dr. A.S. Abraham, containing many of the responsa of R. Shlomo Zalman Auerbach that were otherwise not published)

NARR – New American Reform Responsa (R. Walter Jacob)

NRR – New Reform Responsa (R. Solomon B. Freehof)

R. – Rabbi or *Rav*

RROT – Reform Responsa of Our Time (R. Solomon B. Freehof)

SSK – *Shmirat Shabbat K'hilchata* ("*Observance of the Sabbath According to Its Halacha*" by Rabbi Yehoshua Neuwirth)

Sh Ar - *Shulchan Aruch* (Code of Jewish Law - R. Joseph Caro)

TE – *Tzitz Eliezer* (Responsa of R. Eliezer Waldenberg)

TRR – Today's Reform Responsa (R. Solomon B. Freehof)

ZT"L – *Zecher Tzaddik L'vracha* ("may his righteous memory be a blessing," Hebrew expression used to offer respect to the dead)

# INTRODUCTION

The state of the Jewish world today may be appropriately characterized by a prominent Biblical verse: "See, I place before you today a blessing and a curse...." (*Deuteronomy* 11:26).

On one hand, Jews are living in the midst of the Third Commonwealth, with the independent, democratic State of Israel recently celebrating its 50th anniversary. Peace treaties have been concluded between Israel and Egypt and Jordan, and with the prospect of an agreement with the Palestinians and its other Arab neighbors at hand, Israel is finally assuming a role as the center of world Jewry and has become a leader in technology and science in the Western world and the Middle East. The Jewish people have witnessed the liberation of hundreds of thousands of brethren from Eastern Europe, Ethiopia, and the Arab states, allowing them to immigrate to Israel and other countries to live freely as Jews. In the United States and Western Europe, Jews enjoy a level of acceptance, influence and affluence in society that is unparalleled in history. There has been a renaissance on the part of both men and women in the study of Torah and classic Jewish texts worldwide. It is estimated that there are a greater number of Jewish day schools and *yeshivot* (schools devoted to religious study) in Israel than at any other time. As the ideal of a "melting pot" has gradually given way to recognition of the inherent value of a "mosaic" or "salad", the opportunity exists for Jews outside of Israel to lead religious lives.

On the other hand, the Jewish world is plagued by internal crises that rival the greatest the Jewish people have experienced. The astounding rate of intermarriage, with estimates ranging at levels as high as over 50 percent in the Diaspora, and interdenominational strife over issues of personal status such as "who is a Jew," marriage, divorce and religious conversion in Israel, pose significant threats to the future of the Jewish people from within. As serious and legitimate as these problems are, effective solutions remain elusive while the animus only increases.

This book endeavors to capitalize on the strengths of contemporary Jewish life in order to address some of these issues. It is an effort to demonstrate in tangible terms that Judaism, through its rich legal and ethical tradition, is capable of successfully and meaningfully addressing some of the most difficult problems we face -- particularly those encountered in the realm of medical ethics. For physicians and professionals in particular, this book also attempts to demonstrate the potential for synthesis and harmony between secular and religious life. Just as *Shabbat* (the Sabbath) serves as *me'ein olam haba,* a brief foretaste of the world to come, the application of Jewish medical ethics is a contemporary example of Rabbi Samson Raphael Hirsch's philosophy of "*Torah im derech eretz*" ("Torah and the way of the world").

During the past several years, I have had the opportunity to study Judaism with numerous scholars from around the United States as part of a unique program for community leaders sponsored by the Wexner Heritage Foundation. This experience vastly broadened my Jewish awareness, provided me with exposure to different perspectives, and allowed me to gain an appreciation for the value of a pluralistic approach. As an observant Jew and a general surgeon who has spent the better part of the past two decades focusing on the care of high-risk and often critically ill and injured patients, I have been constantly amazed at the ability of Jewish tradition (i.e., Jewish law - *halacha*) to effectively guide me as I dealt with ethical dilemmas encountered in my own clinical practice. I have always found the Jewish approach to these complex problems to be logical and thoughtful, and displaying a degree of flexibility I never imagined possible. More importantly, I have yet to encounter a situation in which the guidance I received by consulting Jewish tradition led me in a direction or placed me in a predicament in which I felt morally uncomfortable. My confidence in, and appreciation for the accumulated wisdom of our sages and rabbinic decisors continues to grow.

Living in a medium-sized American Jewish community and being a member of the faculty at a prominent medical school has afforded me the opportunity to teach Jewish medical ethics to students, faculty and lay people. As a result, I value education and open-mindedness in bringing Jews closer to Judaism. Specifically, teaching a subject matter such as medical ethics from a Jewish perspective provides Jews of all backgrounds, as well as non-Jews, with an appreciation that Judaism is a *living* religion, culture, civilization and legal system, with an incredibly rich tradition that is interested in and capable of successfully addressing those ethical and moral dilemmas confronting society. Exposure to such personally relevant material has proven to be an effective way to touch people's lives and bring them closer to Judaism.

It is from this perspective, as an observant Jew, surgeon, student and teacher that I have embarked upon this endeavor. Many noted scholars have published works on Jewish medical ethics over the past four decades since the publication of Rabbi Immanuel Jakobovits' seminal work *Jewish Medical Ethics* in 1959. This book is not intended to compete with these works, but rather complement them by incorporating their valuable contributions and presenting them through the use of a novel approach. First, this book is written primarily for people who may lack a strong background in medicine, medical ethics or Judaism. For this reason, I provide adequate introductory and background information in these areas, as well as a glossary of terms to make this topic understandable to the novice (**Part I**). Second, in order to make the subject matter relevant to people's lives and allow them to place the ethical dilemmas into a "real" context, the format of the book differs from others in the field. The ethical discussions and analyses have been presented in the context of a clinical case scenario, depicting the fictitious medical and ethical dilemmas encountered by a patient and her family as they deal with a succession of devastating events (**Part II**). I have made the clinical case medically accurate without being overbearing in its details, yet interesting enough to entice the reader to continue to the end. Third, I have provided a broad spectrum of ethical and legal opinions representing prominent streams of thought within each of the branches of contemporary Judaism. The purpose of this book is to demonstrate that, despite differences between denominations in many other areas of Jewish life and practice, the approach to the resolution of ethical dilemmas in medicine is remarkably similar, employing the same classical texts, sources and reasoning. Additionally, because the book is meant to provide an introduction to the field of Jewish medical ethics, the references cited are not exhaustive. Classic sources are referenced, as are most of the contemporary works in this area that have been published in English. Preference is given to noting references in books over journals because of their availability to a general audience.

Finally, the following disclaimer is in order. I am neither a rabbi, ethicist or Talmudic scholar. The material presented here has been culled from a wide variety of sources and woven together in order to present a coherent body of Jewish thought dealing with ethical conflicts in medicine. Where disagreements between decisors and texts exist, I have attempted to point them out. The purpose of the book is to introduce the subject material through the eyes of Jewish tradition. This book does not purport to present *halacha le'ma'aseh* (practical Jewish law) and nothing in it should be interpreted in that manner. Specific questions dealing with these matters in real life should properly be referred to a trained rabbinic authority for resolution.

I fervently hope that this work will serve as an inspiration to its readers by demonstrating that Judaism and the Jewish tradition remain alive and vibrant after more than 2,000 years; that Judaism is interested and capable of responding meaningfully and responsibly to the most challenging crises of our day; and that Judaism, and the study of the tradition, are indeed relevant to our lives both as Jews and citizens of the world. If any should begin studying Judaism more seriously as a result of reading this book, the effort will have validated itself.

R. Tarfon: It is not incumbent on you to finish the task, neither are you free from beginning it....(Mishnah, *Avot* 2:16)

# Acknowledgments

No endeavor like this is conceived, nor occurs in a vacuum. Numerous people deserve my heartfelt thanks and appreciation for their contributions to this effort. Without their support and assistance, it is doubtful whether this project would have ever even begun. First, my teachers over the last several years from the Wexner Heritage Foundation and the Columbus Community Kollel deserve praise for helping me acquire a deeper and broader appreciation of Judaism and learning. Most notable among them is my teacher, publisher, and friend, Dr. Ronald Brauner, who demonstrated his deep commitment to Jewish outreach and education in the most tangible way by inviting me to write this book. Second, my students, colleagues, and *chevra* from the "basement minyan," whose encouragement and positive reinforcement have spurred me to keep writing, merit attention. Third, my friends, Dr. Paul Pollack, who suggested the title, Dr. Rochelle Millen, Dr. Paul Nelson, and Lori and Jeff Lasday, who gave of their personal time and expertise to read, critique and improve the manuscript. And especially, to Deborah Biskin Levine, who painstakingly read and reread every word of it, and rewrote many parts of it, as well as to my copy editor at Mirkov, Lori Silberman Brauner. *Acharon, acharon chaviv* (last but not least), my family, especially my children, Meir, Shira and Tova, who supported this effort by allowing me the time to read, think and get on the computer every now and then in order to write, deserve gratitude.

# PART I

## Chapter 1: ORIGINS AND DEFINITION OF JEWISH MEDICAL ETHICS

Ethics is the branch of philosophy that studies moral values and judgments. It is concerned with determining the morally correct thing to do in any particular situation, the "rightness" or "wrongness" of an act. In contrast, law defines those actions that are permitted and prohibited by society under various circumstances and the punishment incurred for a transgression. Thus, laws may be ethical or unethical, just or unjust, or morally neutral. A just society seeks to construct an ethical legal system

(Knobel). The use of ethical principles in such a fashion is known as *applied ethics*.

The latter half of the 20$^{th}$ century, in the aftermath of the Second World War, has spawned almost unimaginable technological advances in science and medicine that have enhanced our lives in countless ways. Innovations in medicine have also given rise to a wide array of ethical and moral dilemmas that challenge society as a whole as well as its various constituents -- political, ethnic, racial, religious, professional and gender-based groups, and unaffiliated individuals.

*Biomedical ethics*, or *bioethics*, is a subcategory of general ethics in which standard philosophical principles are applied in the analysis of moral problems and judgments as they specifically relate to clinical medicine, behavioral sciences and biomedical sciences. The field of biomedical ethics began to evolve in the 1960s as issues arose involving the allocation of scarce medical resources such as intensive care unit beds, equipment for hemodialysis, and cadaver organs for transplantation. Interest in biomedical ethics has grown tremendously with the development of scientific and technological advances. The spectrum of ethical concerns addressed in the field of bioethics is almost endless, and includes public health policy and the allocation of health care resources; the integrity and limits of the doctor-patient relationship; personal autonomy, privacy and confidentiality; the proper conduct of medical research involving human and animal subjects; problems associated with reproductive rights and technology; and terminal illness, death and dying. Many of these issues will confront some of us in our own lives.

In general or secular biomedical ethics, numerous principles have been identified which form the basis for analyses. Four of these, respect for autonomy or self-determination, nonmaleficence (do no harm), beneficence (doing good), and justice (equality), have been grouped together as core values and coined the "Georgetown Mantra." Other recognized ethical values that are useful in evaluating dilemmas are paternalism (the notion that "father knows best"), confidentiality, truth-telling, courage, loyalty, and hard work. In recent years, the field of secular medical ethics has been characterized by a dramatic shift in the doctor-patient relationship -- from one of paternalism and beneficence, with the physician at the center of medical decision-making -- to that of autonomy, self-determination and privacy, with the patient as the major or even sole focus of decision-making. The latter approach might be referred to as autonomous ethics. More recently, another shift has occurred from individual or patient autonomy to "unilateral" autonomy, whereby physicians and/or ethicists may make decisions, such as the withdrawal or limitation of care, without the express consent of the patient or his or her family. Central to this analysis in general ethics is the fact that the principles, goals and limits invoked in making choices are based upon humanly initiated theories and ideas.

At the same time, in the wake of the Holocaust -- the darkest period in all of Jewish history during which a third of the Jewish people were annihilated at the hands of the Nazis -- we have witnessed a renaissance in the study of Torah and Jewish culture throughout the world. This unprecedented increase in Torah knowledge and learning, coupled with the prominence of Jews in the biomedical sciences and clinical medicine, has undoubtedly contributed to the interest of Jewish scholars in both the intellectual and practical aspects of biomedical ethics, the area referred to as Jewish medical ethics.

Jewish medical ethics can be defined as the resolution of bioethical problems based upon the application of philosophical principles in a manner that is consistent with the adhered tenets and traditions of Judaism. This can be understood in several ways, which will be described later, but one critical point must be emphasized at the outset. Something "Jewish" is different from something being done by some Jews. Judaism, while certainly not homogeneous, is far from lacking a distinct form. As a religion, culture and civilization, it has a rich and well-defined literary history replete with primary, secondary and tertiary sources. For an action to be worthy of the appellation "Jewish," it must be firmly grounded in Jewish sources and tradition; that is, it must be based in Judaism. Stealing, murder and idol worship are not "Jewish" activities because Jews engage in them any more than one would consider segregation and slavery "American" ideals simply because some Americans supported them.

Throughout history, Judaism has been a law-based religion, with virtually all aspects of life governed by a comprehensive system of laws called *halacha* (literally – the way). *Halacha,* although practically developed and refined by humans, has ultimately been understood as expressing Divine will and wisdom, so that commitments and obligations are ascribed to a higher moral standard and authority (heteronomous ethics) for both individuals and society, as opposed to individual or personal standards or rights (autonomous ethics). The role of *halacha* in Jewish tradition has been so central that all of classical Jewish philosophy and theology have been derived through its analysis and interpretation. This approach contrasts sharply with our understanding of the evolution and role of law in Western societies (especially the United States) since the Enlightenment, in which the philosophy or the underlying critical principles precede the law, not vice versa. For example, in order to pass a law in the U.S. Congress, among other considerations, a majority of legislators must agree on the legitimacy of a particular virtue or moral principle (such as banning the sale of automatic weapons or drugs). Conversely, if a majority does not subscribe to the value, then the law will not be enacted. In the halachic system, the essential elements of the law, such as the prohibition against murder, theft, adultery -- for example -- are primary, as stated in the Torah. The broader ethical and moral lessons and implications of these laws are derived by man based on the assumption that the premises are eternally valid and inviolate because they represent the will and wisdom of God ("The Torah of God is perfect," *Psalms* 19:8).

A less traditional approach to Jewish medical ethics is based on the notion that ethical principles are fundamentally universal and not particularistic. Thus, there can be no actual Jewish medical ethics, per se. However, in order for the wisdom of the Jewish tradition to inform and participate in a genuine and productive dialogue with general ethics, universal ethical principles must be elucidated from the Jewish tradition through its classical sources and then applied to the resolution of ethical dilemmas. Judaism has been credited with providing Western civilization with such a legacy. Well beyond the Ten Commandments and the "Golden Rule," the Torah remains a revolutionary document. By introducing subtle modifications in contemporaneous laws and customs, the Torah, along with its subsequent tradition of rabbinic interpretation, radically transformed the understanding of justice. For example, the Torah banned the popular practice of human sacrifice, implicitly in the story of the binding of Isaac (*Genesis* 22:1-18), and explicitly with respect to worshiping the god Molech (*Leviticus* 20:2-6), and replacing it with animal sacrifices. The doctrine of "…an eye for an eye, a tooth for a tooth..." (*Exodus* 21:24), taken literally in other cultures (Code of Hammurabi), was never interpreted as such in the Jewish tradition. Rather, it was always understood as implying financial remuneration for damages incurred. Similarly, slavery, as a method of civil or criminal punishment, was transformed into a limited form of indentured servitude, and women were granted unprecedented protection in the areas of marriage and divorce. Other such principles include the Seven Noahide laws (prohibitions against idolatry, blasphemy, murder, stealing, adultery, eating the limb torn from a live animal, and the establishment of a civil court system) and virtues such as compassion and charity, which are repeatedly extolled by the Prophets. In these and many other arenas, Judaism and its associated ethical tradition have given the Western world fundamental and now, almost universally accepted, ethical principles.

The difference between the secular and Jewish approaches to biomedical ethics hinges on the differences between ethics and law; the practical implications of these approaches are significant. Secular ethics, employing philosophical analysis, reaches conclusions that are not binding in any enforceable manner. Furthermore, with the current emphasis on individual autonomy as the overarching ethical principle in decision-making in contemporary Western culture, it is difficult if not impossible to arrive at any broad-based societal consensus. Traditional Judaism, on the other hand, utilizes a halachic or legal analysis to resolve ethical dilemmas, resulting in interpretations that become normative and binding on its adherents and, therefore, constitute obligatory behavior. This latter approach is particularly relevant when discussing the views of more liberal denominations of Judaism, which have ascribed more value to the ethical commandments and principles within Judaism than to the ritual obligations. Similar conflicts have arisen over the years between secular ethics and other religious approaches, which are examples of deontological ethics (systems that defer to absolute moral authority, such as God). The differences in the degree and seriousness of the ethical conflicts between Judaism other religions and secular ethics, is a function of the centrality and importance of *halacha* in Jewish life.

## Chapter 2: OVERVIEW OF JEWISH LAW
### (*Halacha* - literally: the way)

Judaism is fundamentally legal in its orientation, with virtually all aspects of life orchestrated by *halacha*. Laws governing human behavior have been the primary focus of Jewish life, providing patterns of conduct for individuals within the family and community. Such laws, dictating a person's manner of speech, integrity in business and fulfillment of communal obligations such as charity, take precedence over non-legal principles. "He has told you, man, what is good and what the Lord requires of you: only to do justice and to love goodness, and to walk humbly with your Lord" (*Micah* 6:8). Our sages have taken the position that the human purpose, or more specifically the task of the Jewish people, is to "perfect the world within the kingdom of God" (*Aleinu* prayer), a task which is accomplished by living a life emulating the Almighty and performing God's commandments (*mitzvot*).

Philosophical and theological principles in Judaism have been considered secondary, derived through the analysis and interpretation of laws. Therefore, it is essential in any discussion of Jewish medical ethics that one possesses a working knowledge of Jewish law. What follows is a brief overview of its development, structure and function.

The primary source from which all of Jewish law is ultimately derived is the *Torah* (Pentateuch, Five Books of Moses, Written Law or *Torah she'bichtav*), which, according to tradition, was "revealed" by God to the children of Israel through Moses at Mount Sinai approximately 1300 BCE. The *Torah* is distinguished from the *Tanach* (canonized Hebrew Bible or Old Testament) which is comprised of the *Torah*, the *N'vi'im* (Prophets) and *K'tuvim* (Writings). The Pentateuch consists of five books: *B'reishit* (*Genesis*), *Sh'mot* (*Exodus*), *Vayikra* (*Leviticus*), *Bamidbar* (*Numbers)* and *Devarim* (*Deuteronomy),* and contains 613 commandments (*mitzvot*) that obligate Jews in an array of tasks governing the relationship between human beings and God (*bein adam lamakom*) and between one person and another (*bein adam lachaveiro*). Certain commandments dealing with ritual matters are not applicable in contemporary society since their performance requires the use of the Temple (which no longer exists). Examples of such practices include the laws of animal sacrifices, priesthood, and ritual purity and defilement. These 613 commandments have also been categorized as 248 positive commandments (*mitzvot asei*), which prescribe certain actions, and 365 negative commandments (*mitzvot lo ta'aseh*), which prohibit other actions. Among these *mitzvot* are those that seem logical and could be derived by humans, such as not stealing or murdering, which are called *mishpatim*. Other commandments, for which there is no logical explanation, such as the laws of ritual purity, are termed *chukim*.

In the Jewish tradition, the Written Law is accompanied by the Oral Law (*Torah sheb'al peh*), which expounds on specific commandments and provides explanations concerning their precise implementation. This is not unique to ancient Judaism, since most legal codes in existence at the time of the Torah (and even to our own day) have had oral traditions associated with them. In classic Jewish belief, the Oral Law and the principles for interpreting it were given to Moses on Mount Sinai at the time the Torah was revealed. It was sequentially passed on to Joshua, Aaron, and the Elders, who in turn transmitted it to the Prophets and eventually to the Rabbis, through the time of the destruction of the Second Temple in the year 70 CE, and into the Babylonian exile . [This sequence of transmitting the *mesorah* (religious heritage) is delineated at the beginning of the *Ethics of the Fathers* (*Pirkei Avot*) and in Maimonides' introduction to his *Commentary on the Mishnah* and *Mishneh Torah*].

The Oral Law comprises several categories of legislation: (1) laws whose explanations were given by Moses, that are derived from the Torah; (2) *halacha l'Moshe miSinai* (laws given to Moses at Mount Sinai); (3) laws that are derived through logical reasoning, but about which there may be differences of opinion; and (4) rabbinic legislation, which consists of *takanot* (rabbinic enactments) and *g'zeirot* (rabbinic decrees). All of these forms of rabbinic legislation carry the force of law, based upon the text of the Torah (*Deuteronomy* 17:9-11): "You shall come to the…judge [rabbi] who will be in those days; you shall inquire and they shall tell you the word of judgment. You shall do according to the word that they will tell you, that they will teach you. You shall not deviate from their instructions to the right or to the left."

The first category of Oral Laws consists of laws whose explanations are believed to have been given directly by Moses and passed down through the generations. They are grouped together because their explanations are either hinted at or can be logically derived from the text of the Torah. These laws have traditionally been accepted by all Jews without disagreement. Examples from this category include such items as who is required to dwell in a *sukkah* (booth) and the knowledge that the fruit of a *hadar* tree (*Leviticus* 23:40) is an *etrog* (citron) and that of the *avot* and *arvai nachal* are myrtle and willows.

*Halacha l'Moshe miSinai* are laws believed to have been transmitted directly from God to Moses and then from Moses through the generations as described above, although there is no logical explanation that can be related to the Torah text. They carry the legal weight of Written Law. Maimonides, in his Mishneh Torah, enumerates thirty examples of *halacha l'Moshe miSinai* that include such things as the manner of construction of *t'fillin* (phylacteries), the minimum sizes and measures used for certain rituals and specific technical requirements for writing a Torah scroll.

The largest group of Oral Laws contains those laws derived by analysis and logical reasoning. It is about these laws that disputes among decisors arose which are recorded in the Talmud. The Talmud is the written version of the Oral Law, compiled over a period of five centuries.

Around the year 200 CE, Rabbi Judah the Prince (also known as *Rebbe* and *Yehuda HaNasi*), head of the *Sanhedrin* (Chief Court) and the most respected sage at that time, committed the Oral Law to writing, fearing that it was being eroded and would be lost over time. His redaction, known as the Mishnah (to study), is written in Hebrew and consists of six divisions called *sedarim* (orders), which, in turn, are further subdivided into 63 *masechtot* (tractates). In general, the Mishnah simply reports the law without reiterating the elaborate discussions of the Rabbis of the period (called *tannaim*).

Over the next three centuries, academies of Jewish learning in Babylon and Palestine primarily studied the Mishnah to elucidate the intricacies of Jewish law. In the fifth century, 400-500 CE, sages in Babylon and Palestine (referred to as the *amoraim*) committed their extensive commentaries on the Mishnah, known as the Gemara, to writing, collectively called the Babylonian and Palestinian or Jerusalem Talmud. The Jerusalem Talmud was composed by Rabbi Yochanon around 400 CE and contains 50 tractates. The Babylonian Talmud was compiled by Rav Ashi and Ravina about 500 CE. Written in Aramaic, it consists of 35 tractates and is generally considered the more authoritative of the two. The tractates correspond and expound upon those in the Mishnah. Many tractates of Mishnah have no Gemara associated with them, presumably because the discussions in the Babylonian academies did not focus on every aspect of law, especially those addressing Temple ritual and the land of Israel. The *Talmud* consists of two general types of material – *halacha* (legal practice) and *aggadata or aggada* (non-legal discussions offering moral and historical teachings and observations). The halachic portions of the Talmud were derived using a series of rules of exegetical interpretation employing texts, inference and analogy, which allow legal comparisons to be made and judgments to be drawn. The best known of these are the "13 *middot* (hermeneutical principles) of R. Ishmael," which are still employed today in halachic analysis. From this point onward, the Talmud has been considered the fundamental corpus of Jewish law.

Rabbinic legislation also includes pronouncements, called *takanot* and *g'zeirot*. *Takanot* are rabbinic enactments that are usually designed to impose a duty to perform some act, in order to preserve harmony among people and promote Torah observance. Examples of *takanot* still in force are the requirement to read *megillat Esther* (scroll of Esther) on the holiday of Purim and the lighting of Chanukah candles. G*'zeirot* are decrees based upon the Biblical verse "Safeguard my charges" (*Leviticus* 18:30), whose purpose is to prevent certain actions or "make a fence" (*siyag*) around the Torah to avoid any possible violation of Biblical commandments. Examples of "fences" that have been constructed around the law include rabbinic restrictions against "work" on *Shabbat* and the prohibition against eating poultry (which was technically *pareve*, neither meat nor dairy) with dairy products in order to avoid any possible violation of the laws of *kashrut* by confusing poultry with meat.

Some rabbis of the Talmud composed additional texts to assist in the elucidation of the Torah and the Mishnah, known as *midrashim*. *Midrashim* consist of legal (halachic) and homiletic (aggadic) commentaries on the *Tanach* which "fill in gaps" in the story line, providing explanations of complexities in the text. *Mechilta, Sifra, Sifre* (halachic *Midrashim*) and *Midrash Rabbah* and *Midrash Tanchuma* (aggadic *Midrashim)* are among the better-known works.

The period of time following the redaction of the Talmud until the 10th century, known as the Gaonic period (*Gaon* was the title of the head of a major Babylonian academy), saw the introduction of several important tools to enhance the understanding and teaching of the Torah and Talmud. These included *perushim* (elucidative commentaries), codes of law, *she'eilot u'tshuvot* (questions and answers or responsa), as well as *takanot*, *g'zeirot* and additional *midrashim.*

*Perushim* have been grouped chronologically, according to the commentator. The earliest commentators after the Geonim, referred to as *Rishonim* (the "first ones"), composed their commentaries before the appearance of the *Shulchan Aruch* (Code of Jewish Law), while *Achronim* (the "later ones"), wrote commentaries that succeeded the *Shulchan Aruch.* The pre-eminent Biblical and Talmudic commentator is R. Shlomo ben Yitzchak (known as Rashi), who lived in the 11th century. Other early commentators on the Talmud include the Tosafot, a group of 12th- and 13th-century scholars, R. Moses ben Nachman (known as Nachmanides, Ramban), and R. Nissim Gerondi (referred to as the Ran).

The first attempts to codify, and thereby organize and clarify the vast array of legal material contained in the Talmud also occurred during the Gaonic period. The Middle Ages, characterized by the dispersion of the Jewish people, saw further creations of codes of Jewish law. The earliest of these was written by R. Moses ben Maimon (known as Maimonides, Rambam), a 12th-century physician and philosopher. Entitled the *Mishneh Torah* or *Yad HaChazakah,* this 14-volume, topic-oriented opus was the Rambam's attempt to simplify and summarize all of Jewish law to date. The next major code, the *Arba'a Turim* or *Tur*, was compiled by R. Jacob ben Asher in the 14th century. Divided into four sections based upon the four rows of the *Kohen Gadol's* (High Priest) breastplate, the *Tur* has served as the template for all subsequent codes. The sections are entitled: *Orach Chayim*--laws of prayers, Sabbath and festivals; *Yoreh Deah*-- laws of forbidden and permitted foods, vows and purity; *Even HaEzer*--laws of marriage, divorce and sexual relations; and

*Choshen Mishpat*--civil and criminal law, inheritance and property. The *Tur* served as the authoritative code until the 16th century, when the *Shulchan Aruch* ("set table"), by R. Joseph Caro, supplanted it. The *Shulchan Aruch*, based upon the structure of the *Tur*, is actually a Sephardic (Jews originating from the Iberian Peninsula) document. Shortly after its publication, R. Moses Isserles (known as the Rama) added a gloss, referred to as the *Mappah* ("tablecloth"), depicting the corresponding Ashkenazi (Continental European Jewry) practices. These works have remained the dominant code of Jewish law. Several codes have since been published to update or clarify the laws in the *Shulchan Aruch* and *Mappah*, most notably the *Aruch HaShulchan* by R. Yechiel M. Epstein in the 19th century and the *Mishnah B'rurah* by R. Israel Meir HaCohen (known as the Chafetz Chaim) in the early 20th century.

The final category of Jewish law consists of customs (*minhagim*) and practices, which differ from *halacha* in that their legitimacy results from their popularity among the inhabitants in a particular geographic area. The importance of *minhag* was appreciated early in Jewish tradition. "Do not abandon the customs of your ancestors" (JT, *Pesachim* 4:1). "The custom of your ancestors is Torah" (Sh Ar, *Yoreh Deah* 376:4). "Never deviate from custom. When Moses ascended on high, he ate no bread nor drank (*Exodus* 34:28), and when the angels came down to earth, they ate bread and drank (*Genesis* 19:3)" (BT, *Bava Metzia* 86b), meaning that when Moses was among God and the angels, he did not eat or drink because they did not, and when the angels visited Abraham and Sarah, they ate and drank with them. Over time, *minhagim* assume the status of law and can serve either to fill a gap in existing law where no specific provisions exist to address a particular problem or to resolve a dispute in its interpretation. In certain circumstances, a *minhag* may even override existing law, termed *minhag mevatel halacha.* The significance given to *minhagim* is perhaps the best example of Jewish tradition's recognition of pluralism within its ranks. Variations in *minhag* and *nohaig* are respected and accepted as legitimate differences; this is Judaism's version of "more than one way to skin a cat." Examples of this are the variations in ritual techniques, eating habits and liturgy among Ashkenazim, Sephardim and Chassidim. For example, some Ashkenazi men do not wear a *tallit* (prayer shawl) before marriage, whereas Sephardim and some Ashkenazim do. There are also differences in the technique of putting on *t'fillin* and the liturgical texts and sequence of the prayers. Also, different groups wait varying periods of time between eating meat and milk.

Despite the availability and authority of the codes of Jewish law, legal codes cannot anticipate and address every conceivable situation. Thus, the predominant form of perpetuation and interpretation of Jewish law in the modern era (post-1800) has been *she'eilot u't'shuvot* (rabbinic responsa to specific questions), a practice popularized during the Gaonic period that continues today. The collections of rabbinic "case law" generated over centuries have provided the richest source of material for use in solving ethical dilemmas.

In this vein, a number of contemporary *poskim* (rabbinic decisors) have made major contributions in the area of Jewish medical ethics. Some of the important Orthodox thinkers in this area include Lord Immanuel Jakobovits, who was formerly the Chief Rabbi of the British Commonwealth and is considered the "Father of Jewish Medical Ethics." In the United States, Rabbi Moses Feinstein, zt"l (1895-1986), recognized as the pre-eminent halachic authority in the world during his lifetime and author of *Iggrot Moshe,* published many *t'shuvot* dealing with medical ethics. Other American authorities include Rabbi Dr. Moses Tendler, son-in-law of Rabbi Feinstein and a respected biologist and halachic decisor in his own right, and Rabbi Dr. J. David Bleich, perhaps the most widely published and respected Orthodox spokesman on Jewish bioethics in the United States. Both Tendler and Bleich are on the faculty of Yeshiva University. In Israel, Rabbi Shlomo Zalman Auerbach, zt"l (1910-1995) was recognized as one of the pre-eminent halachists of this generation. Rabbi Eliezer Waldenberg, author of the *Tzitz Eliezer*, is the most prominent and prolific living Israeli halachic decisor in this area. In addition, Rabbi Chaim David HaLevy, z"tl, the former Sephardic Chief Rabbi of Tel Aviv, and Rav OvadiaYosef, the former Sephardic Chief Rabbi of Israel, have issued a number of influential rulings in the area of medical ethics and *halacha*. Members of the Conservative movement who have made significant contributions to our understanding of Jewish medical ethics include Rabbi David Feldman, who authored several of the earliest and most authoritative English-language texts in this area, and Rabbis Elliot Dorff, Aaron Mackler, Avram Reisner and Joel Roth, who have also written extensively on this subject matter. The Reform movement has published numerous responsa over the years dealing with topics in medical ethics. Most of these were composed by Rabbis Solomon Freehof and Walter Jacob.

In addition to these prominent rabbinic scholars, several physicians with recognized expertise have made significant contributions to this field. In the United States, Fred Rosner, M.D., an internist, is the foremost English- language author in the area of Jewish medical ethics. Rosner has also translated a number of Maimonides' medical works into English. In Israel there are several major figures. Avraham S. Avraham, M.D., an internist, has written several halachic works in Hebrew dealing with Jewish medical ethics, *Lev Avraham* and *Nishmat Avraham.* Avraham Steinberg, MD, a pediatric neurologist and rabbi, has published numerous books and articles, most notably the *Encyclopedia Hilchatit U'Refuit*. Mordechai Halperin, MD, an obstetrician-gynecologist and rabbi, has also published widely in this field. These individuals will be cited repeatedly throughout this book; without their contributions, the field of Jewish medical ethics would not have developed as it has.

Familiarity with the various texts that have been written over the course of Jewish history is critical for readers of this book, but they also need to become acquainted with the halachic process itself. Utilizing the halachic process for contemporary ethical (or other) issues involves several basic steps. Initially, one must seek and identify legal precedents, often via inference or analogy, from classic Jewish sources (Torah, Talmud, midrash, codes, responsa, etc.) and then adduce the underlying principles. These precepts must then be applied to each new set of facts. This process, as in any established legal system, is highly structured and follows well-defined rules that govern the interpretation of texts and application of specific principles, thereby developing new law.

The Jewish legal system is hierarchical, with "authority" flowing from the divine downward. This is based upon the premise that each succeeding generation is less worthy than the previous one, which was chronologically closer to the revelation at Mount Sinai. Thus, in Jewish law, the highest level of authority is the Torah (*d'oraita* in Aramaic), followed by that of the Talmud (*d'rabbanan* in Aramaic), with primary Torah laws superseding Talmudic or rabbinic laws. Together, the Torah and Talmud can be understood as forming the statutory basis of all Jewish law. Based upon this schema, the opinions of *Tannaim* (rabbis from the Mishnaic period) take precedence over those of *Amoraim* (rabbis of the *Gemara*). Similarly, in terms of commentators (such as

Rashi, Tosafot, Ramban, etc.), codes of Jewish law (*Mishneh Torah, Shulchan Aruch, Aruch HaShulchan* and *Mishnah B'rurah*), and responsa, which serve as precedents in the Jewish legal tradition, those authored by *Rishonim* generally take precedence over those of *Achronim*. Nonetheless, the principle of *hilchata k'vatra'ai*, "*the law is according to the* later authorities" very often applies. While elements of the halachic process are universal, disagreements among authorities within a given branch of Judaism exist or arise because of differences involving selection, interpretation and application of textual sources. Such divergent opinions have existed and been recognized as part of the halachic system within rabbinic Judaism since its inception, as evidenced by the inclusion of minority opinions in the Talmud. The Talmud (BT, *Eruvin* 13b), in describing the clashes between the House of Hillel and the House of Shammai, validates various viewpoints by stating: "These and these are the words of the living God." In another passage (BT, *Chagigah* 3b), in response to a question about how one can learn Torah from scholars in the midst of widespread disagreement, the Talmud justifies such arguments by stating: "All of them are given from one Shepherd." Similarly, conflicting visions between streams of Judaism or within one group occur because of variations in assumptions made regarding the applicability of Jewish law and sources.

Just as contention arises within the Jewish legal system, gaps are also manifested between Jewish and secular law. This was especially true after the Emancipation, as Jews began integrating into society and the ability of the religious community (*kehilla*) to govern itself in matters of civil law declined. Since then, matters of civil law within the Jewish community have largely been superseded by the civil laws of the host country based on the principle (a *takanah*) of *dina d'malchuta dina* (the law of the land is the law – derived from *Nehemiah* 9:37). It is only in matters of marriage, divorce and other issues of personal status that *halacha* has continued to function parallel with civil law.

## Chapter 3: RELIGIOUS DENOMINATIONS IN CONTEMPORARY JUDAISM

The current system of Jewish law, generally referred to as Rabbinic Judaism, originated during the Talmudic period after the destruction of the Second Temple. This methodology and structure persisted as the legacy of the Pharisees, as other sects within Judaism, such as the Sadducees, Qumran community and even early Hebrew-Christians, disappeared or evolved into separate religions. Rabbinic Judaism continued generally unchallenged (with notable exceptions among the Karaites, Sabbateans and Frankists) from within as the dominant mode governing Jewish life until the Enlightenment and Emancipation in the mid-18$^{th}$ and 19$^{th}$ centuries. At this juncture, in the late 18$^{th}$ century, Reform Judaism was founded in Germany as an attempt to facilitate acculturation and discourage the assimilation of the Jewish community in Germany. Reform Judaism soon spread to the New World, where it was readily accepted and enjoyed considerable popularity. At the turn of the 20$^{th}$ century, an immigrant wave of more traditionally practicing Jews from Eastern Europe brought what is now referred to as Orthodox Judaism to the United States. Shortly thereafter, in an attempt to find a middle ground for Jews in America, some traditionalists founded what is now known as Conservative Judaism. Finally, Reconstructionism arose as an outgrowth of Conservative Judaism in the mid-20$^{th}$ century.

These branches vary significantly in their practice of Judaism. The discrepancies in religious behavior are the result of basic differences in their understanding and interpretation of several key elements within Judaism. Below follows a brief summary of the approach of each of these movements to a number of core components of Jewish thought and praxis: the existence of God, the nature of Revelation, the nature of the Torah and Oral Law and the role of *mitzvot* and humans in the evolution of Jewish law.

**Orthodox Judaism**. Orthodox Judaism considers itself the heir to traditional Judaism as it has been practiced since Talmudic times. Orthodoxy maintains that God exists as creator, ruler and controller of the universe. Revelation at Mount Sinai was a singular event with direct communication from God to Moses and the people of Israel, during which the Torah was given. The Torah is God's will and word, verbatim, as dictated to and recorded by Moses. The Oral Law was also conveyed expressly by God to Moses at Mount Sinai, and was transmitted verbally and eventually written down as the Talmud. All the *mitzvot* are binding and obligatory as they represent the explicit will of God. Qualified rabbinic authorities can reinterpret the law by applying specific rules to deal with contemporary issues and problems. Orthodoxy insists upon the primacy of the verse: "You shall not add to the word that I command you, nor shall you subtract from it....," (*Deuteronomy* 4:2, also *Deuteronomy* 13:1). Practically speaking, according to Orthodox belief, all commandments that are capable of being performed are still obligatory.

In Orthodox Judaism, there is no central body or legal authority to dictate matters of *halacha*. All ordained rabbis have the prerogative to decide issues of Jewish law. The weight given to a particular individual's halachic decision by his peers and the community is dependent upon that rabbi's standing as a scholar and *posek* (rabbinic decisor). For this reason, complex issues that arise in disciplines such as medical ethics are specifically referred to individuals with such recognized expertise.

Although the principles governing the role and development of Jewish law within Orthodoxy are standard, the Orthodox Jewish community is hardly monolithic in its approach to legal complexities. Orthodoxy has been colloquially subdivided into segments that span a spectrum of opinion from right-wing, ultra-Orthodox and hasidic sects to more modern, centrist or left-wing Orthodox camps.

**Conservative Judaism**. Conservative Judaism contains a spectrum of opinion about the nature and role of God, but all of its prominent thinkers believe that God exists and plays a role in the unfolding of the universe and the course of history. Revelation did occur at Mount Sinai, consisting of direct communication between God, Moses and the people of Israel. However, revelation has also been experienced at other times throughout history and continues in our own time (continuous revelation), depending upon our ability to perceive and comprehend it. The Torah is a Divinely inspired document representing human interpretation and understanding of God's will, but is not necessarily a verbatim accounting of God's word. Similarly, the Oral Law represents human interpretation of God's law as well as ongoing custom and law dating back from even before the Revelation at Mount Sinai. *Mitzvot* are still binding and obligatory because they represent God's will and because they have been upheld as authoritative by the Jewish community historically and in own own time. It is natural for our understanding of God's wishes to evolve over time, and change is an evolutionary, not revolutionary, process. Thus, qualified rabbis can reinterpret and change Jewish law because the historical context of Biblical times is not necessarily reflective of our own (positive historical approach). In this context, the Rabbis in each generation have the specific responsibility to reinterpret the law because of our ongoing understanding of our relationship with God. This approach is grounded in the weight that Conservative Judaism gives to the several key Biblical verses dealing with the interpretation of law. "You shall come to the .....judge [rabbi] who will be in those days; you shall inquire and they shall tell you the word of judgment. You shall do according to the word that they will tell you, that they will teach you" (*Deuteronomy* 17:9-10).

Rashi quotes the Talmud (BT *Rosh Hashanah* 25a-25b) in commenting on this verse. He states that "in those days" implies that the authority of the contemporary rabbis is binding, even if they are of lesser stature than those of previous generations. "Surely this instruction which I give you today is not too baffling for you, nor is it beyond reach. It is not in the heavens, that you should say 'Who among us can go up to the heavens and get it for us, and get it for us and impart it to us that we may observe it?" (*Deuteronomy* 30:11-12). This verse charges the people with the interpretation of the law, by declaring that it is no longer in heaven (also BT, *Bava Metzia* 59b). From a practical standpoint, all commandments that can be performed at present are still binding unless the rabbinic leaders of a particular generation determine that there is some overriding reason why they should not be.

Decisions of Jewish law within the Conservative movement are made more formally than within Orthodoxy. The Rabbinical Assembly, in cooperation with the seminaries of the Conservative movement and the United Synagogue of Conservative Judaism, maintains an active Committee on Jewish Law and Standards that makes determinations concerning *halacha* for the Conservative movement. However, only when the Committee's decision is adopted as a standard of the movement is its decision binding on all rabbis and adherents of Conservative Judaism. When a decision is instead adopted as a valid position, each rabbi has the prerogative to resolve the matter for him/herself, using the opinions expressed by the Committee in an advisory manner.

**Reconstructionist Judaism**. An outgrowth of Conservative Judaism, Reconstructionism is the child of Rabbi Mordecai M. Kaplan. Kaplan believed that God, as a discrete or supernatural entity, does not exist. Rather, God represents "the power that makes for salvation, that is, the creative power in nature and the one that makes for goodness. God thus serves as a "guiding light" throughout life. Since God is not personal, Revelation could not have occurred. Instead, Judaism should be understood as a complete "religious civilization" evolving from Biblical times to the present, with its own unique laws, customs, folklore, art, music and language. The Torah, written by men, describes God's will (universal, guiding moral and ethical principles) as they understood it. The Oral Law, in turn, reflects human opinion at the time it was composed. Ethical *mitzvot* are considered to represent God's will and should serve as guiding principles by which to live. Ritual *mitzvot* reflect the ideas and rulings of the prophets and rabbis in their times, and are no longer binding upon us. Since it is recognized that ritual *mitzvot* are important in preserving tradition and transmitting values, their observance is encouraged and valued. However, it is the responsibility of individuals and congregations to make the appropriate decisions regarding issues of ritual practice. In terms of changing law, the Rabbis of each generation have the responsibility to interpret and modify laws and traditions as they see fit for the betterment of the community.

**Reform Judaism**. Reform Judaism acknowledges that God exists; however, there is disagreement about whether God actually created and currently controls the world. Some Reform thinkers believe that some kind of revelation between God and Israel occurred, but its precise characterization is unclear, and that revelation continues to this day as our understanding of God's will evolves (progressive revelation). The Torah was written by men, based upon their understanding of God's will. Similarly, the Oral Law represents human analysis of the laws of the Torah as they were understood during Talmudic times. For this reason, ritual *mitzvot* are felt to represent the opinions and rulings of the prophets and rabbis in their times, and because these rituals may not be relevant today, these *mitzvot* are no longer binding or in force.

Furthermore, the Reform movement has eliminated all vestiges or references to the ancient Temple service from its liturgy as well as the traditional classification of personal status, *Kohen, Levi* and *Yisrael.* Although observance is entirely up to the individual, Reform Jews recognize that ritual *mitzvot* may be useful in preserving the tradition and transmitting certain values, and recent Reform platform statements (1976, 1999) urge Reform Jews to learn as much as possible about Judaism so that they make their own autonomous choices about Jewish ritual with knowledge rather than in ignorance. The ethical *mitzvot,* however, are considered eternally valuable as guiding principles in life, and are therefore binding, in the tradition of the prophets.

Although *halacha* is not binding for Reform Jews, the Central Conference of American Rabbis has a Committee on Bioethics that has addressed a number of controversial areas affecting Jewish life and issued position papers to guide its constituents.

It has become commonplace in discussions involving differences between religious denominations and matters of Jewish law to place Orthodox Judaism at one extreme, the Conservative Movement in the middle and the Reconstructionist and Reform Movements at the other. However, in dealing with a subject such as medical ethics, it may be more useful to separate them based upon their views regarding the role of *halacha.* In such a classification, Orthodox and Conservative Judaism would be grouped together because each considers *halacha* binding, while Reform and Reconstructionism do not.

There is only one *Torah*, one *Talmud*, one *Mishneh Torah*, one *Shulchan Aruch*, with a common halachic methodology employed. Thus, in analyzing a particular ethical or halachic dilemma, members of various movements refer to the same classical sources. However, similarity in process does not guarantee singularity in outcome. Because of their differing assumptions and understanding of the history and structure of Jewish law, they will often reach conflicting conclusions. In most cases, Jewish law may be viewed as a continuum, from the strictest interpretations (Orthodox) to the most liberal interpretations (Reform). Where one stands on the continuum regarding a specific situation is a function of the perspectives and degrees of weight that any rabbinic decisor places on the specific source material and precedents analyzed.

Unfortunately, it is inevitable that not all issues in bioethics have been addressed by each of the current movements. However, guidelines to anticipate the approaches that each would take can be formulated based upon their respective views of Jewish law. Generally, issues that are permissible according to Orthodox authorities are allowed by more liberal denominations. Conversely, issues that are forbidden according to more liberal denominations will also be forbidden by the Orthodox. Disagreement usually arises in those situations that are permitted by more liberal branches, but are not necessarily deemed permissible by the more traditional movements.

# PART II

## CLINICAL CASE SCENARIO

*The Chollims are a religiously observant Jewish family. Mara and Chaim Chollim have been married for 26 years. They have 4 children, Naomi (23 years old), Benjamin (20 years old), Devorah (17 years old) and Rafi (11 years old). Naomi and Benjamin are their biological children, Devorah and Rafi, who are biological siblings, were adopted after their parents died in an accident. Naomi, Benjamin and Rafi are in excellent health.*

*Devorah has had brittle diabetes mellitus since early childhood. She has been hospitalized numerous times from complications, including diabetic ketoacidosis (an emergency arising from the blood sugar being out of control), pneumonia and urinary tract infections. She missed a significant amount of school, which was especially difficult during her college preparatory years, and is discouraged and depressed because of her worsening health problems. She has a poor social life and is becoming increasingly withdrawn. During Devorah's early adolescence, she was meticulous about her diet and exercise regimen. However, as she entered young adulthood, she has become resentful that her disease sets her apart from her peers. She is rarely invited to the movies or to parties with her friends. On the rare occasions that she does participate in activities with her classmates, she avoids any social situations that involve eating. She is embarrassed that she cannot share pizza, french fries or ice cream with her friends.*

*As a result of her isolation and loneliness, she has begun to rebel and exhibit self-destructive behavior. She disregards her diet and has stopped checking her blood sugar regularly, causing her to experience insulin reactions, such as hypoglycemia (low blood sugar) or hyperglycemia (elevated blood sugar) with ketoacidosis. Her parents and older siblings feel that they need to be more involved in her day-to-day management and care.*

*As any young adult, Devorah desires more autonomy and independence. Her family's increased interference in her life makes her act in a more belligerent manner. She has become distrustful of her physicians and her entire health care team because her condition continues to get worse despite her having carefully followed her prescribed treatment regimen.*

*Neither Devorah nor her family can understand how or why this is happening to them. They are good, honest, God-fearing people. Why are they being punished and made to suffer like this? They consult their rabbi for advice.*

*Devorah is angry about her family's increased incursion into her life and begins to behave rebelliously, plotting to deter them. She creates obstacles to the observance of the Sabbath, when certain categories of "work" are prohibited. For example, Mara shops and prepares meals on Thursday night for Shabbat. When her mother's back is turned, Devorah throws the food into the garbage; by the time Mara goes to serve meals on Friday evening, she discovers that the food is gone. The lack of a proper meal creates problems for the entire family since cooking and shopping are prohibited on the Sabbath, but especially for Devorah, since her diet is restricted. On several occasions, Devorah's improper eating has necessitated trips to the emergency room.*

***Four months later.*** *Devorah is experiencing more complications of her diabetes. She has begun manifesting signs of gastroenteropathy (difficulty with digestion and movement of the stomach and intestines, causing pain and constipation), worsening* *eyesight, peripheral neuropathy (numbness and loss of sensation in her legs) and the onset of renal (kidney) dysfunction. Her doctors believe that this progression could be slowed or even halted if her diabetes were under better, "tighter," control. They discuss the possibility of two experimental treatments: the transfer of pancreatic islet cells (the cells in the pancreas that are responsible for the manufacturing and secretion of insulin into the bloodstream for the digestion of sugar), or an injection of a genetically engineered virus that could produce human insulin. Although, the chances that either of these will be successful is only between 10 and 20 percent, success would lead to dramatic improvement in her condition, perhaps even a "cure." Viewing this treatment as a "quick fix," Devorah's attitude becomes a bit more positive.*

*However, Devorah's parents and grandparents, as Holocaust survivors, are especially skeptical of any "medical research" because of the way the Nazis conducted "experiments" on Jews, Gypsies and other prisoners of war. Just hearing the term "medical research" sends chills up their spines. It brings back horrible memories for them, particularly Devorah's grandfather -- himself a subject of the Nazis. Much consultation with their rabbi and Devorah's physicians is necessary to help everyone make this difficult decision. The fact that Devorah suddenly feels so optimistic about this procedure helps motivate her parents to offer their consent.*

*Devorah's family is finally convinced that it is reasonable to attempt an Islet cell transfer. However, her insurance carrier, a managed care company, refuses to authorize the treatment because it is experimental. The family begins a lengthy appeal process, but to no avail. The company refuses to give in and cover the procedure and she must forego it. Understandably, Devorah is disappointed, yet decides to persevere with the assistance and support of her family.*

***Six months later.*** *Devorah requires frequent admissions to the hospital. Her renal failure has progressed and she now needs hemodialysis treatments three times a week. She has become depressed and despondent to the point of being suicidal, and does not want to continue dialysis. Once, when she was home alone, she took an overdose of pills which, while ultimately harmless, demonstrated her intention to end her life and suffering. She is often at odds with her family and health care givers as they insist that she continue treatment. She has begun incessantly drinking* *and smoking cigarettes, even marijuana. These indulgences, which further impair her health, are a chronic source of strife between Devorah and her family. She feels that this is the one small aspect of her life over which she still has some control. A psychiatrist is consulted.*

***Eight months later.*** *Because the long-term survival of diabetics on dialysis is poor, doctors recommend that Devorah undergo a kidney transplant, which would offer her a better chance for survival and potentially, a more "normal" lifestyle. Living related donors are preferable because their organs offer a greater chance of long- term success. As Devorah's only living blood relative, Rafi, a minor, is the only potential organ donor available. He, however, is afraid of doctors and hospitals, and has expressed doubts about the potential risks posed to him.*

*Rafi's attitude places Mara and Chaim in an untenable position. Do they encourage one child to potentially endanger his health in order to save the life of his sister? They are angry and resentful that they are confronted with these impossible decisions. Rafi cannot help but feel guilty that he is not stepping forward more eagerly to assist his older sister. But, having watched her suffer in the past, he does not want to find himself in a similar position later in life.*

*After observing his sister suffer and deteriorate over time, Rafi eventually consents to becoming an organ donor. However, the medical team reconsiders and feels that a combined pancreas-kidney transplant might be a better long-term treatment option because it could possibly "cure" her diabetes and stop the progression of her complications. Devorah and her family agree for her to undergo a combined pancreas-kidney transplant. Rafi's soul searching and meritorious gesture become moot because a pancreas cannot be taken from a living donor. She is placed on the waiting list for a cadaver transplant.*

***Four months transpire.*** *A serious motor vehicle accident occurs. The victim is a 34-year-old Jewish male, Natan. He has suffered a severe head injury due to blunt trauma along with a lung contusion and pelvic fracture. His condition is critical and after he is initially stabilized in the emergency department, he is transferred to the intensive care unit (ICU) for further care. His condition worsens over the next 48 hours and his physicians believe that his head injury will be fatal. They inform his family, initiate an evaluation for neurological or brain death, and notify* *the organ procurement network and transplant team. The next morning, Natan is pronounced "dead, based upon neurological criteria," and his family is approached about the possibility of organ donation. Although Natan checked off the organ donor box on his driver's license, his family's consent is still required. They quickly consult their rabbi about this difficult decision.*

*Natan's family agrees to the organ donation. The kidney and pancreas are successfully transplanted into Devorah, and the heart, lungs, liver and corneas are sent elsewhere for transplantation. She does well following the transplant and is discharged for home after two weeks.*

***Six months later.*** *Devorah's life dramatically improves. Again, she is committed to following carefully all of her doctor's orders. She takes her medications with great care. After recovering from surgery, she begins a new job. She would like to begin dating, but is very self-conscious about her appearance. Her self-esteem was badly damaged through her adolescent years and she has little confidence or experience in social situations. She wants to have a rhinoplasty ("nose job"), which she believes will improve the way she looks, and consequently, her self-esteem and social life. Devorah's parents are skeptical about any additional* *surgery, even elective surgery. They feel as though she has already "been through enough."*

***Two months later.*** *Devorah undergoes a rhinoplasty. She feels better about herself and begins dating. After a few months, she meets and falls in love with a nice young man, Gabriel. Gabriel is willing to marry Devorah despite all of her medical problems. However, his parents are concerned about her illness and long-term prognosis. They would like to discuss her medical problems with Devorah's physicians. Devorah is resentful about this intrusion into her private affairs. She feels strongly that these issues are personal, or only between Gabriel and herself.*

***One year later.*** *Devorah and Gabriel marry. After a year, they contemplate starting a family. They discuss this with Devorah's doctors, who voice concern about the stress of pregnancy on Devorah and the chances of her children developing diabetes or some other genetic problems because of the immunosuppressive medications she is taking. The situation is further complicated because there is a questionable history of Tay-Sachs disease (a uniformly fatal, genetically transmitted disease that affects Ashkenazi Jews) in Gabriel's family. The doctors are highly skeptical and advise them to postpone children for awhile* *because of their fear that pregnancy could exacerbate Devorah's medical condition and compromise the viability of her transplant. The couple is advised to utilize birth control in the meantime; the doctors have even suggested that they contemplate sterilization.*

*Devorah does not want to see any child of hers suffer as she has. However, all of her friends are having babies and she feels that she does not want to miss experiencing pregnancy and motherhood. She is constantly sad and cannot get the idea of having a baby out of her mind.*

*Devorah and Gabriel's circumstances appear to have calmed down and stabilized. After a year, they are still interested in having a child. They finally obtain permission from her physicians, although with much reluctance. Unfortunately, it is difficult for Devorah to conceive because of her diabetes and numerous medications. Gabriel is willing to consider adoption, but Devorah is obsessed with the idea of having a biological child. She wants to finally do something "normal" in her life. The couple, particularly Devorah, are anxious to pursue advanced methods of infertility treatment to assist with conception.*

***Eight months later.*** *Devorah undergoes artificial insemination with Gabriel as the donor and eventually conceives.*

*An ultrasound examination early in the pregnancy suggests that there may be four fetuses. Devorah's obstetrician feels that it will be too risky for her to try to carry all of them to term and suggests aborting two or three. Although Devorah would never consider abortion under normal circumstances, she accepts the doctor's advice while trying not to let the pain she feels about aborting these fetuses interfere with the joy she feels from carrying her own baby. She is beginning to believe that things are finally starting to "go her way." The couple is interested in having an amniocentesis performed and trying to select a boy and a girl.*

*Two of the fetuses are successfully aborted at random and the pregnancy continues. However, in the fourth month, Devorah is admitted to the hospital with signs of toxemia of pregnancy (hypertension, renal dysfunction, glucose intolerance). The doctors are worried that she could lose her transplanted kidney and pancreas and recommend that the pregnancy be terminated. At first, Devorah refuses to submit to an abortion. Gabriel, her parents, in-laws, siblings and physicians try in vain to convince her. Gabriel is devastated and tries to convince Devorah that he cannot go on living without her.*

*Devorah reluctantly undergoes a therapeutic abortion, but her condition continues to worsen. She understands that there is a reasonable chance that she may die from the complications of her illness. Suddenly she summons all of the emotional strength she has left and expresses interest in preparing an advanced directive.*

*Devorah develops severe pneumonia with acute respiratory failure, requiring her to be placed on a mechanical ventilator. Her renal function worsens to the point that her kidney transplant fails and she again needs hemodialysis. She is experiencing considerable discomfort and asks her family if she can be "put out of her misery." By the time they mention this to her doctors, she is unconscious. Her condition is grave and her doctors are beginning to lose hope. They inform the family about Devorah's grim outlook and initiate a discussion about establishing limits for treatment. Gabriel and Devorah's parents begin to feel that as her condition deteriorates her doctors are less available to them. They are angry, hurt and feel abandoned by the professionals they have come to count on over the years.*

*Devorah's status continues to decline. After extensive deliberations, the decision is made to withhold further aggressive treatment. A week later, Devorah is allowed to die. The doctors are unsure why Devorah's condition deteriorated so rapidly. They are concerned that she may have developed an unusual fatal infection that could affect other transplant patients. In the hope that an examination of Devorah's body could provide important new information that could help them care for other transplant patients, they ask permission to perform an autopsy. Gabriel and Devorah's parents are offended by this request, feeling that it is insensitive and poorly timed.*

*Devorah's parents are devastated and brokenhearted by her death. They devoted most of their lives to caring for their sick child and, just as they were hoping that she could begin to have some semblance of a normal life, she was taken from them. They are disgusted by what they perceived to be the callousness with which Devorah and they were treated near the end of her life. In addition, they have begun questioning whether closer prenatal care and follow-up could have prevented this final series of complications. Finally, they are quite shocked and overwhelmed at the magnitude of the medical bills for her care, especially since she died despite treatment. For all of these reasons, they are contemplating a medical malpractice lawsuit.*

## Chapter 4: ROLES AND RESPONSIBILITIES

*The Chollims are a religiously observant Jewish family. Mara and Chaim Chollim have been married for 26 years. They have 4 children, Naomi (23 years old), Benjamin (20 years old), Devorah (17 years old) and Rafi (11 years old). Naomi and Benjamin are their biological children, Devorah and Rafi, who are biological siblings, were adopted after their parents died in an accident. Naomi, Benjamin and Rafi are in excellent health.*

*Devorah has had brittle diabetes mellitus since early childhood. She has been hospitalized numerous times from complications, including diabetic ketoacidosis (an emergency arising from the blood sugar being out of control), pneumonia and urinary tract infections. She missed a significant amount of school, which was especially difficult during her college preparatory years, and is discouraged and depressed because of her worsening health problems. She has a poor social life and is becoming increasingly withdrawn. During Devorah's early adolescence, she was meticulous about her diet and exercise regimen. However, as she entered young adulthood, she has become resentful that her disease sets her apart from her peers. She is rarely invited to the movies or to parties with her friends. On the rare occasions that she does participate in activities with her classmates, she avoids any social situations that involve eating. She is embarrassed that she cannot share pizza, french fries or ice cream with her friends.*

*As a result of her isolation and loneliness, she has begun to rebel and exhibit self-destructive behavior. She disregards her diet and has stopped checking her blood sugar regularly, causing her to experience insulin reactions, such as hypoglycemia (low blood sugar) or hyperglycemia (elevated blood sugar) with ketoacidosis. Her parents and older siblings feel that they need to be more involved in her day-to-day management and care.*

*As any young adult, Devorah desires more autonomy and independence. Her family's increased interference in her life makes her act in a more belligerent manner. She has become distrustful of her physicians and her entire health care team because her condition continues to get worse despite her having carefully followed her prescribed treatment regimen.*

*Neither Devorah nor her family can understand how or why this is happening to them. They are good, honest, God-fearing people. Why are they being punished and made to suffer like this? They consult their rabbi for advice.*

This introductory scene raises several questions about the roles and responsibilities of God, patients, physicians and clergy in various aspects of illness and healing. While all of these do not pose ethical dilemmas per se, they are important and challenging questions that people, especially members of a faith community, naturally ask and seek answers to.

**Issues:** Judaism's view of the role of God in illness and healing

Obligation of patients to undergo treatment

Role and responsibility of physicians in healing

Beneficence, paternity and autonomy

Role of the rabbi in medical decision-making

## Judaism's View of the Role of God in Illness and Healing

Nothing tests the faith of believers more than the sight of an innocent child, like Devorah, suffering. Understanding the role of God in sickness and health is not a simple matter. *Theodicy* is the defense of God in the face of the existence of evil or suffering in the world, a subject that has been debated by Jewish and non-Jewish philosophers and theologians throughout the ages without resolution. "It is not in our hands to explain either the tranquility of the wicked or the affliction of the righteous" (*Mishnah*, *Avot* 4:18). Nevertheless, it is appropriate to begin any study of Jewish medical ethics with such a discussion.

Judaism is built upon a covenantal relationship between God and Israel that entails shared responsibilities, mutuality and reciprocity, which carry positive and negative consequences. Fundamental to this belief system is the existence of a God who is concerned with the lives of human beings and is omnipotent, omniscient, perfectly just and merciful. The first of Maimonides' 13 Principles of Faith states: "I believe with perfect faith that the Creator, blessed be He, creates and directs all of His creations, and He, Himself, does, did, and will direct all actions." The commentator Rashi explains, in the first verse of *Genesis* (1:1), that it was originally God's intention that the world be governed exclusively by the divine attribute of justice. However, it became immediately apparent that human imperfection made this impossible; hence the use of two terms for the Divine name (*Elokhim* for the attribute of justice and *YHVH* for mercy).

The problem of theodicy arises because it does not appear that Divine justice and mercy always prevail, raising several troubling questions. If God is all-powerful and merciful, then is God unjust because evil exists? If God is fair and merciful, then is God simply incapable of preventing evil in the world? Or, if God is all-powerful and just, then does the existence of evil imply that God does not care? Each of these queries has been addressed in Jewish tradition.

The earliest references to the doubting of God's justice are in the Torah. Both Abraham and Moses engage the Almighty in dialogues questioning God's judgment. In *Genesis* (18:23-25), Abraham argues on behalf of the inhabitants of Sodom and Gomorrah asking, "Will you indeed destroy the righteous with the wicked?.... It will be sacrilege to you. Shall not the judge of the earth do justly?" Later, after God told Moses that God would decimate the children of Israel following the sin of the spies in the desert, Moses pleaded: "Then Egypt, from whose midst You delivered this nation with your power, will hear and they will say that....you killed this people like a single man....because Hashem lacked the ability to bring this people to the land that He had sworn to give them, He slaughtered them in the wilderness..." (*Numbers* 14:13-16). Thus, there is a strong Jewish tradition of the righteous questioning and arguing with God.

These passages raise the issue of the existence and origins of evil in a world supposedly controlled by a God that is all good, all-powerful and merciful. Does evil come from God? Did God create evil and if so, for what purpose? The classical response is that evil does not and cannot come from God, who is perfect. "Nothing evil dwells with God" (*Midrash Psalms* 5:7), "Evil does not descend from above," "God's work is perfect, for all God's ways are judgment" (BT, *Bava Kamma* 50a), and "Everything God does is for the good" (BT, *B'rachot* 60b). This approach leads to the inevitable conclusion that, since evil cannot emanate from God, it must come from human beings. Humans are capable of evil because God has granted them free will, affording them the option of exercising that liberty. If humans choose to sin, then justice, in the form of Divine retribution, will be administered. This paradigm of reward and punishment is documented throughout the Torah:

> "But if you will not listen to me and will not do all these commandments....I will even appoint over you terror, consumption and fever, that shall consume the eyes and cause sorrow of heart." (*Leviticus* 26:14-16); "It will be that if you listen to my commandments that I command you today, to love Hashem your God and to serve him with all of your heart and with all of your soul, then I shall provide rain for your land....and you will eat and you will be satisfied. Beware, lest your heart be seduced and you turn astray and serve other gods.....the wrath of Hashem will blaze against you; He will restrain the heaven so there will be no rain, and the ground will not yield its produce and you will be swiftly banished from the land that Hashem gives you..." (*Deuteronomy* 11:13-17); and "And also every sickness and every plague, which is not written in the book of this Torah, will the Lord bring upon you, until you are destroyed." (*Deuteronomy* 28:61).

The Talmud (BT, *Shabbat* 55a) extends this concept further, espousing the position that "There is no death without sin, no suffering without transgression." Similarly, we are taught, "For there is no righteous person on earth who does good and will not sin" (*Ecclesiastes* 7:20). Nachmanides, a 12th-century philosopher and physician wrote, "It is proper for any person who has suffered a mishap or some evil experience to believe that his accident and trouble are the result of his transgression and sin...." These pronouncements, however, need not be taken literally and do not necessarily imply that sickness and suffering constitute Divine retribution for conventional transgressions against God or other people. Rather, they may be signs of personal failures or indiscretions in caring for oneself. We are charged to "be exceedingly heedful of yourself" (*Deuteronomy* 4:15) and that "the soul that I have placed inside you, you must give it life and sustain it" (BT, *Ta'anit* 22b). Failure to adequately care for one's health will inevitably result in illnesses and perhaps even premature death. The Jerusalem Talmud (*Shabbat* 14:3) states that 99 out of 100 premature deaths are the result of negligence. Maimonides agrees that the most frequent source of "evil" befalling man is self-inflicted [*Guide for the Perplexed* (3:12)], and not an act of Divine retribution or punishment.

We have all encountered situations in which the punishment does not seem to fit the "crime." In these circumstances, several traditional explanations for Divine retribution have been offered. One explanation is that certain individuals may suffer for the sins of others or the entire people of Israel may be punished for the sins of a few. This is highlighted in Jewish liturgy, most poignantly in the *Musaf* service for festivals ("Because of our sins were we exiled from our land....") and the *kinot* (lamentations) recited on *Tisha B'Av* (the ninth day of the month of Av, corresponding to the destruction of the First and Second Temples in Jerusalem, 586 BCE and 70 CE). This concept has also been presented positively: "All of Israel is responsible one for the other" (BT, *Shevuot* 39a). Alternatively, punishment for sins in the present ("this world," *olam hazeh*) may be a spiritual cleansing or opportunity for repentance, in preparation for redemption and entry into the messianic era and the world to come (*olam haba*). "For whom the Lord loves, the Lord rebukes, as father the son whom he favors" (*Proverbs* 3:12). Experiencing such *yisurim shel ahavah* (afflictions of love), analogous to the contemporary colloquialism "no pain, no gain," actually brings humans closer to God. Rabbi Shimon bar Yochai stated that hardships are precious because

Israel received three precious gifts through experiencing affliction: the Torah, the land of Israel, and the world to come (BT, *B'rachot* 5a). Finally, the Talmud's exhortation (BT, *B'rachot* 5a) that one "analyze one's deeds to determine the cause of suffering" does not necessarily imply that suffering represents punishment. Rather, it can be viewed as an opportunity to improve oneself.

Unfortunately, none of these explanations adequately addresses the suffering of the righteous. With the belief that a higher purpose was to be found from one's suffering, the Rabbis introduced the idea of delayed gratification into the tradition. What appears to be reward for the wicked actually represents their "payoff" in this world because true happiness and reward will come in the messianic era and the world to come. "In this world we see the godless prosper and the faithful suffer. There must, therefore, be another world in which all will be recompensed in justice and righteousness" (Saadia Gaon, *Emunot v'deot*). "There is no reward for fulfillment of the precepts in this world" (BT, *Kiddushin* 31b). "In this world the righteous are smitten, but in the World to Come they will have firm footing and strength" (*Midrash Psalms* 1:20).

Postulating the existence of a world to come does not resolve the dilemma of *why* God allows the righteous to suffer or evil to exist. In the Bible, this is most dramatically portrayed in the book of *Job*, in which Job, who is "blameless and upright, who feared God and shunned evil," is severely punished by God for no apparent reason. Job confronts God, but never loses faith. The response God eventually gives to Job (Chapters 38-41) is that God rewards and penalizes people for their actions and controls history. God is just and things do happen for a reason, but it is beyond the realm of humans to understand God's ways. Ultimately, Job is vindicated and rewarded for his unyielding faith in the face of adversity. God's response to Job is similar to that which God gave to Moses following the sin of the Golden Calf, when he asked: "Let me behold Your glory!" And He answered, "I will make all My goodness pass before you....and I shall show favor when I choose to show favor and I shall show mercy when I chose to show mercy.... you cannot see My face, for man may not see Me and live....Then I will take My hand away and you will see My back; but My face must not be seen." (*Exodus* 33:18-23).

This issue is especially perplexing in the 20th century following the Holocaust. No satisfactory answer can or does exist.

Several explanations have been proposed, ranging from the classic responses of Divine retribution and the incomprehensibility of the ways of God to the more radical ideas that God must be dead (Richard Rubenstein) and that the covenant with the Jewish people has been severed forever (Irving Greenberg). Many of us with close connections to the Holocaust and its victims find one or more of these proposals troubling, if not completely unpalatable.

The Talmud (BT, *Shabbat* 55b) also recognized an inconsistency in the classic approach to suffering and evil: "There is death without sin and suffering without transgression." This statement, especially if applied to illness, is consistent with Maimonides' view of the existence of evil in the world, as expressed in his *Guide for the Perplexed* (3:12). Here, Maimonides describes three causes of evil in the world. Although he subscribes to the view that sin results in retribution and people often contribute to their own misery, Maimonides recognizes that only by having the choice to do good or evil can man appreciate good. Maimonides explains that bodily decay, illness and death are natural components of the human condition, which is consistent with the Talmudic declaration: "The world pursues its natural course...." (BT, A*vodah Zarah* 54b). The implications of this approach are profound, as it offers a way to accept illness and suffering in a traditional light without invoking blame and guilt on the individual or God.

Viewing illness as a natural component of life instead of Divine retribution allows one to approach God and ask for mercy and healing. The idea that God plays a role in healing is introduced in the Torah (*Exodus* 15:26): "If you will diligently listen to the voice of the Lord thy God, and will do that which is right in His sight, and will listen to His commandments and keep all His statutes, I will put none of these diseases upon you which I have brought upon Egypt; for I am the Lord that heals you." Such a plea for God's assistance in curing illness has been incorporated into the liturgy. In the *Avinu Malkeinu* prayer, we say, "Our Father, our King, send complete healing to the sick of your people" and in the weekday *Amidah*, "Heal us God--then we will be healed; save us--then we will be saved, for You are our praise. Bring complete recovery to all our ailments, for You are God, King, the faithful and compassionate healer. Blessed are You, God, who heals the sick of His people Israel."

Much in Jewish tradition contributes to the paradox concerning the respective roles of God and human beings in the genesis and healing of human disease. If illness represents a Divine decree promulgated on mankind, and it is, in fact, God who heals illness, how then can one administer or pursue medical treatment and remain faithful to God?

## Obligation of Patients to Undergo Treatment

Based upon the preceding discussion, one who is ill must seek treatment or else risk Divine retribution. Jewish tradition recognizes the need and obligation for individuals to seek medical attention, based upon the notion that we are responsible for our bodies while on earth. The Tanach acknowledges the role of physicians in several places. Joseph employs house physicians (*Genesis* 50:2), Isaiah refers to the services of a surgeon (3:7), and King Hezekiah is ultimately praised for destroying the *Book of Treatments* written by King Solomon (described in Mishnah, *Pesachim* 4:9).

More specifically, the Torah contains several admonitions concerning each individual's responsibility to care for himself, according to Rabbinic tradition: "Take heed of yourself, and take care of your life" (*Deuteronomy* 4:9); "Take exceedingly good care of your lives" (*Deuteronomy* 4:15); "When you shall build a house, you shall make a railing around the roof, that you shall not bring blood upon your house if any man fall from there" (*Deuteronomy* 22:8). Similar exhortations appear in the Talmud: "A man should not place himself in danger" (BT, *Shabbat* 32a); and "Whoever is in pain, let that person go to the physician" (BT, *Bava Kamma* 46b). The importance of having access to health care is upheld by the prohibition against a scholar to live in a town without a physician (BT, *Sanhedrin* 17b).

Additional evidence for the justification to seek medical attention is presented in the *Midrash* (*T'rumah 2*):

> R. Ishmael and R. Akiva were walking through the streets of Jerusalem with another man. They met a sick man who asked: "Masters, how may I be cured?" They replied: "Do such and such and you will be cured." After the sick person left, the man accompanying them asked: "Rabbis, who afflicted him?"
>
> "The Holy One, Blessed be He," they answered.
>
> A bystander then interjected: "You interfered in a matter which is not your concern. God afflicted him, why do you wish to heal him?" The Rabbis asked him: "What

> is your vocation?" "I am a tiller of the soil. Here is the scythe in my hand," he answered. The Rabbis then inquired: "But who created the vineyard?"
>
> "The Holy One, Blessed be He," he said.
>
> "Then you interfered in this vineyard which is not yours? He created it and you cut away its fruits?" asked the Rabbis.
>
> "Do you not see the scythe in my hands? Were I not to go out and plow and till and fertilize and weed, the vineyard would not produce any fruit," the farmer explained.
>
> They said: "Fool, from your own work you have not learned that it is written (*Psalms* 103:15): 'As for man his days are as grass.'" Just as the tree, if not weeded, fertilized and ploughed will not grow and bring forth its fruit...so it is with the human body. The fertilizer is the medicine, the healing is the means, and the tiller of the earth is the physician.

A contemporary source for allowability to seek medical attention can be based upon the interpretation of *Genesis* 1:28 by R. Joseph B. Soloveitchik in his essay *The Lonely Man of Faith*:

"....be fruitful and multiply; fill the earth and subdue it, and rule over the fish of the sea, the birds of the sky and every living thing that moves on the earth." The obligation to "subdue it, and rule over [it]..." empowers us to seek medical assistance. If God has seen fit to allow mankind, modern medicine and science to develop advanced treatments for disease, then it is entirely appropriate, indeed mandatory, that we utilize them. Thus, in this view, seeking medical treatment constitutes the fulfillment of God's wishes. This is consistent with the Talmud's understanding of the role of human action in the face of danger: "In danger, one must not rely on miracles" (BT, *Kiddushin* 39b); and "Never depend on a miracle" (BT, *Shabbat* 32a). The implication of these warnings is clear: one does not know when, if or how the Almighty will intervene, and therefore, one must do whatever one can to preserve life under adverse conditions.

Having established a religious mandate to seek medical attention, the parameters of that requirement must be delineated. For example, is it an absolute requirement to seek and accept medical treatment for all problems and under all circumstances? Are minor ailments and serious or terminal conditions considered equal? Do mitigating circumstances, such as the degree of pain and suffering, matter? Is there room for personal choice or autonomy? From whom should treatment be sought? Should preference be given to Jewish physicians?

The answers to these questions are complex and vary depending upon each specific situation. Several of these issues will be discussed in greater detail as the clinical history unfolds. At this juncture, some basic guidelines can be introduced.

Medical treatments are divided into two broad types, those about which the efficacy is known (*refuah bedukah*) and those where the efficacy is unproven (*refuah she'einah bedukah*). Examples of *refuah bedukah* are conditions such as appendicitis, for which surgery is curative; infections like pneumonia or a strep throat, which are treated with antibiotics; abscesses that require drainage, or fractures that must be reduced and casted. Medical attention for non-emergent conditions, such as pregnancy, are also examples of *refuah bedukah* because the benefits of prenatal care have been well-documented. In these types of cases, most authorities have opined that a Jew is obligated according to *halacha* to undergo treatment. These judgments are based on the principle that life is precious and we are required, as custodians of our bodies, to care for them. In order to do so, we are obligated to utilize those means that God has provided (or allowed to be developed) for that purpose.

Alternatively, one is not required to undergo a *refuah she'einah bedukah.* In these cases, regardless of whether there are potential risks involved, since the results of the treatment are unproven, the halachic onus placed on the patient is reduced and the patient is given greater autonomy.

According to the late Rabbi Feinstein, the standard employed in Jewish law to define the success of a treatment is a greater than 50 percent chance of achieving a cure or restoring the patient to functional health, not that of persistent pain and suffering. A cure is defined as more than one year's duration of life (*chaye olam*), as opposed to a moment of life (*chaye sha'ah*). These definitions do not require that a guarantee of a cure be made or achieved because it is well-recognized that a cure is not always possible. "With regard to cures, there is naught but danger; what heals one kills another" (Nachmanides, as quoted by *Beit Yosef, Tur*, 336).

Regarding the choice of physicians, patients should seek out the most qualified physician for treatment (BT, *Shabbat* 32a). There is no specific obligation to use a Jewish or religiously observant doctor. The only caveat is that one is forbidden to be treated by a physician who proselytizes or promotes heresy.

**Role and Responsibility of Physicians in Healing**

Just as patients are required to seek and receive medical treatment, so too must physicians heal. Justification for human intervention against illness is derived from several sources. The Torah states: "And if men quarrel and one smite the other with a stone or with his fist and he not die but must keep in bed...he must pay the loss entailed by absence from work and cause him to be thoroughly healed" (*Exodus* 21:18-19). From the statement "and cause him to be thoroughly healed," (Hebrew: *v'rahpoh yerapeh*; literally: and heal he shall heal), the Talmud (BT, *Bava Kamma* 85a) deduces that the duplication of the term "heal" implies that the physician is granted license to heal and the patient is authorized to undergo medical treatment. The scope of the medical treatment covered by this verse is fairly comprehensive, and includes payment for five components: physician fees and medical bills, time off from work, shame due to disfigurement, pain and suffering, and physical damage incurred.

The authorization to heal was later extended to an obligation. Maimonides bases this on a different verse: "And you shall restore it to him" (*Deuteronomy* 22:2). Although this sentence actually refers to the return of lost property, Maimonides interprets it as including the restoration of health. This is codified by Maimonides in his *Commentary on the Mishnah* (*Yebamot* 4:4) where he states: "It is obligatory from the Torah for the physician to heal the sick and it is included in the explanation of the Scriptural phrase 'and you shall restore it to him,' meaning to heal his body." Similarly, the Talmud (BT, *Sanhedrin* 73a) states that this verse implies that one "must save his neighbor from the loss of himself."

Others utilize additional Biblical and Talmudic sources to document this obligation, such as "Neither shall you stand idly by the blood of thy fellow" (*Leviticus* 19:16). This negative commandment is one of several duties enumerated by the Torah in *Leviticus* 19, defining a person's behavior toward others. Fundamental moral principles governing human society have been expounded by the Talmud and Maimonides as follows: "Whence do we know that if a man sees his neighbor drowning or mauled by beasts or attacked by robbers, that he is bound to save him? From the verse "Neither shall you stand idly by the blood of thy fellow"

(*Sanhedrin* 73a) and "Whoever is able to save another and does not save him transgresses the negative commandment, 'Neither shall you stand idly by the blood of thy fellow'" (MT, *Hilchot Rotzeach* 1:14). Furthermore, R. Caro (Sh Ar, *Yoreh Deah* 336) posits: "The Torah gave permission for the physician to heal; moreover, this is a religious precept and is included in the category of saving life; and if a physician withholds his services it is considered as shedding blood." Lastly, Nachmanides uses the Biblical verse "And you shall love your neighbor as yourself" (*Leviticus* 19:18) to establish this obligation. Thus, the mandate and requirement for a physician to heal is broad, encompassing four *mitzvot* -- three positive and one negative. This differs from American civil law and the AMA Code of Medical Ethics, which allows physicians an element of choice concerning which patients to treat, but forbids abandonment of patients once they have received treatment (AMA Code of Medical Ethics, 8.11.1997).

A contemporary example of the halachic obligations of physicians to their patients and to society relates to the issue of physician strikes. A major physician strike occurred in Israel in 1983 that spanned several months. During the strike, a number of rabbinic authorities, including R. S.Z. Auerbach and Chief Rabbis

Avraham Shapira and Mordechai Eliyahu, became involved and issued responsa concerning the permissibility of physicians to strike. Uniformly, the opinion of the rabbis was that it was forbidden for physicians to withhold necessary treatment from any patient or to place patients at risk by not providing adequate staffing (defined as the minimum necessary for coverage on *Shabbat*). Although some decisors recognized the legitimate concerns and rights of physicians to receive appropriate compensation, striking was not felt to be an appropriate venue to redress these grievances.

There is a distinction between the halachic obligation for a doctor to heal and any requirement to become a physician. No one is bound to study medicine or become a physician, regardless of how intelligent or talented he or she may be. However, once one becomes a physician, he or she is committed according to Jewish law in all the requirements incumbent upon a practitioner of medicine.

Controversy exists over whether a *Kohen* (priest) is permitted to study medicine. There is a Biblical injunction against a *Kohen* becoming ritually defiled by coming into contact with a dead body (*Leviticus* 21:1-2). Because cadaver dissection is required in medical school and there is no obligation for anyone to study medicine, most contemporary Orthodox authorities, such as R. Feinstein, R. I. Jakobovits, R. J.D. Bleich, prohibit a *Kohen* from doing so. A more lenient view allowing *Kohanim* to study medicine has been advocated by a minority of *poskim*. These opinions are based upon the arguments that the ban against ritual defilement is no longer applicable because there is no method available for ritual purification; furthermore, these individuals will use their knowledge for saving lives, earning a living and healing the sick. The Conservative rabbinate has sanctioned *Kohanim* studying medicine if they "strive to avoid" ritual defilement from dead bodies (CJLS 1927-70, Responsa *Yoreh Deah* 373, p 1444).[1] For Reform Jews, this is a non-issue, since the special personal status of *Kohanim* is no longer recognized.

Having established that physicians have both permission and obligation to heal the sick, it is necessary to address the precise role of the physician in healing. Is it in fact the doctor who heals, or is

---

1. Rabbi Elliot Dorff, in a private communication, informs me that he "doubts that we would now even mention the need for *kohanim* who are physicians to 'strive to avoid' ritual defilement from dead bodies, especially since that is, in practice, impossible in a hospital setting. What they do to save life and health takes precedence over the concern of *toharah* in any case."

it God who heals with the physician functioning as a Divine agent or emissary? Several responses to these questions have been recorded, most notably, those of Ben Sira (*Ecclesiasticus* 38) and Maimonides (*Medical Oath* and *Physician's Prayer*), as follows [as translated in Isaacs, RH. *Judaism, Medicine and Healing.* Jason Aronson, Inc., Northvale, NJ 1998].

**Ben Sira's words:**

Honor a physician before need of him
Him also has God appointed
From God the physician gets wisdom
And from a king he shall receive gifts.
And he shall stand before nobles
God brings out medicines from the earth
And let a prudent man not refuse them.
Was not water made sweet with wood
For to acquaint every man with His power?
And He gave man understanding
To glory in His might.
By them does the physician assuage pain
And likewise the apothecary makes a confection,
That His work may not fail

Nor health from among the sons of men.
My son, in sickness be not negligent
Pray unto God, for God will heal.
Flee from iniquity, and from respect of persons
And from all transgressions cleanse your heart,
Offer a sweet savor as a memorial
And fatness estimated according to your substance
And to the physician also give a place
And he shall not remove, for there is need of him likewise,
For there is a time when in his hand is good success.
For he too will supplicate to God
That God will prosper to him the treatment
And the healing, for the sake of his living.
He that sins against his Maker
Will behave himself proudly against a physician.

### *Medical Oath Attributed to Maimonides*

Your eternal providence has appointed me to watch over life and health of Your creatures. May the love of my art actuate me at all times, may neither avarice nor miserliness, nor thirst for glory, or for a great reputation engage my mind, for the enemies of truth and philanthropy could easily deceive me and make me forgetful of my lofty aim of doing good to Your children.

May I never see in the patient anything but a fellow creature in pain. Grant me strength, time, and opportunity always to correct what I have acquired, always to extend its domain, for knowledge is immense and the spirit of man can extend indefinitely to enrich itself daily with new requirements.

Today he can discover his errors of yesterday and tomorrow he can obtain a new light on what he thinks himself sure today. O God, You have appointed me to watch over the life and death of Your creatures, here I am ready for my vocation and now I turn to my calling.

**Maimonides' *Daily Prayer for the Physician***

Almighty God, You have created the human body with infinite wisdom. Ten thousand times ten thousand organs have You combined in it that act unceasingly and harmoniously to preserve the whole in all its beauty -- the body, which is the envelope of the mortal soul. They are ever-acting in perfect order, agreement, and accord. Yet, when the frailty of matter or the unbridling of passions deranges this order or interrupts this accord, then forces clash and the body crumbles into the primal dust from which it came, You send to man diseases as beneficent messengers to foretell approaching danger and to urge him to avert it.

You have blessed Your earth, Your rivers, and Your mountains with healing substances; enable Your creatures to alleviate their sufferings and to heal their illnesses. You have endowed man with the wisdom to relieve the suffering of his brother, to recognize his disorders, to extract the healing substances, to discover their powers and to prepare and to apply them to suit every will. In Your eternal presence You have chosen me to watch over the life and health of Your creatures. I am now about to apply myself to the duties of my profession. Support me, Almighty God, in these great labors that they may benefit mankind, for without Your help not even the last thing will succeed. Inspire me with love for my art and for Your creatures. Do not allow me thirst for profit, ambition for renown and admiration, to interfere with my profession, for these are the enemies of truth and of love for mankind and they can lead astray in the great task of attending to the welfare of Your creatures. Preserve the strength of my body and of my soul that they be ever ready to cheerfully help and support rich and poor, good and bad, enemy as well as friend. In the sufferer let me see only the human being. Illumine my mind that I recognize what presents itself and that it may comprehend what is absent or hidden. Let it not fail to see what is visible, but do not permit it to arrogate to itself the power to see what cannot be seen, for delicate and indefinite are the bounds of the great art of caring for the lives and health of Your creatures. Let me never be absent-minded. May no strange thoughts divert my attention at the bedside of the sick, or disturb my mind in its silent labors, for great and sacred are the thoughtful deliberations required to preserve the lives and health of Your creatures.

Grant that my patients have confidence in me and my art and follow my directions and my counsel. Remove from their midst all charlatans, and the whole host of officious relatives and know-all nurses, cruel people who arrogantly frustrate the wisest purposes of our art and often lead Your creatures to their death.

Should those who are wiser than I wish to improve and instruct me, let my soul gratefully follow their guidance; for vast is the extent of our art. Should conceited fools, however, censure me, let love for my profession steel me against them, so that I remain steadfast without regard for age, for reputation, or for honor, because surrender would bring to Your creatures sickness and death.

Imbue my soul with gentleness and calmness when older colleagues, proud of their age, wish to displace me or to scorn me or disdainfully to teach me. May even this be of advantage to me, for they know many things of which I am ignorant, but let not their arrogance give me pain. For they are old and old age is not a master of the passions. I also hope to attain old age upon this earth, before You, Almighty God! Let me be contented in everything except

> in the great science of my profession. Never allow the thought to arise in me that I have attained sufficient knowledge. For art is great, but the mind is ever expanding. Almighty God! You have chosen me in Your mercy to watch over the life, and death of Your creatures. I now apply myself to my profession. Support me in this great task so that it may benefit mankind, for without Your help not even the least thing will succeed.

These documents strongly support the concept that physicians are highly skilled actors, assisting the Almighty in a drama in which only God knows the outcome.

**Beneficence, Paternity and Autonomy**

Conflict between the virtues of beneficence and paternity against personal autonomy highlights one of the major areas of disagreement between Jewish tradition and contemporary societal values. Over the past few decades in Western societies, personal autonomy has emerged as the pre-eminent ethical consideration in medical decision-making. Consistent with the American ideal of rugged individualism, this has repeatedly been reaffirmed by the courts in decisions like Griswold v. Connecticut, Rowe v. Wade (1973), Quinlan (1976), Bouvia (1986), Cruzan (1988), and most recently the upholding of the constitutionality of the Oregon Death with Dignity Act (1998).[2]

The benefits of championing personal autonomy have been widely recognized and hailed. However, dramatic shifts in values to the virtual exclusion of any consideration for the rights of society have raised concerns on the part of many Jewish and non-Jewish secular ethicists and theologians. Judaism places extreme value on life as a commodity because human beings were created "*b'tselem Elokhim*" (in the image of God, *Genesis* 1:27). The Talmud (BT, *Sanhedrin* 37a) states: "....Therefore, only a single human being was created in the world, to teach that if any person caused a single soul to perish, Scripture regards him as if he had caused an entire world to perish; and if any human being saves a

---

2. Griswold v Connecticut – established a First Amendment right of privacy that is protected from government intrusion; Rowe v Wade - affirms both a woman's right to privacy and to undergo an abortion; Quinlan - allowed patient in persistent vegetative state to be disconnected from ventilator in accordance with her wishes and those of her family; Bouvia - affirmed the right of a terminally ill patient to refuse a feeding tube; Cruzan - allowed nutrition and hydration to be withheld in accordance with the previously articulated wishes of the patient; Oregon Death with Dignity Act - allows physicians to dispense prescriptions for lethal doses of drugs to terminally ill patients for the purpose of suicide.

single life, Scripture regards him as though he had saved an entire world." Life is viewed as a gift from God and humans are given custody over their bodies while alive, having a responsibility to care for and protect them. People do not own their bodies, nor do they have unrestricted license to do with them as they please. Therefore, Judaism prohibits tattoos and other types of bodily disfigurement (*Leviticus* 19:27-28; 21:5).

Judaism has always recognized that God granted humankind free will. The corollary to this view is that the choice must be governed by parameters set by God and interpreted by the sages, that is, *halacha*. Thus, tension exists between the will of the individual and the limitations placed upon the individual's choice by Jewish law.

Lord Immanuel Jakobovits, former Chief Rabbi of Great Britain, summarizes several of the principles elucidated so far as follows: (1) It is a religious obligation to protect human life and health, incumbent upon a doctor as upon any other person in a position to do so. (2) A doctor is therefore never morally entitled to withhold or withdraw his services, whether or not a contractual relationship exists between him and his patient, unless a more competent doctor is available. A refusal to render medical aid where required is deemed as tantamount to shedding blood. (3) A patient has no right to refuse medical treatment deemed essential by competent medical opinion for the preservation of his or her life or health, and his or her consent need not be procured for such treatment. (4) In the discharge of the doctor's obligation to save life and limb, and in the absence of the patient's consent, the doctor may even be required to expose himself to the risk of legal claims for unauthorized "assault and battery." (5) While the patient should always be informed of treatments and procedures to be applied, both as a matter of respecting rights and to secure cooperation, prior consent is required, and should be sought, only in cases of a) high risk treatments, b) doubtful or experimental cures, and c) differences of opinion among equally competent medical experts. (6) The onus of choosing between various alternative forms of medical treatment, or none at all, rests upon the doctor, and patients should never be expected to render what are *purely medical decisions*. However, in the instance of the availability of reasonable medical alternatives, patient choice is called for.

There will be numerous examples of discrepancies between autonomy and beneficence and paternity (represented by the *halacha*). The manner in which Jewish tradition has approached and resolved these dilemmas will be examined in an attempt to formulate some general guidelines that can be applied in similar situations.

## The Role of the Rabbi in Medical Decision-Making

As ritual and moral conduct in Judaism are governed by statutes, it falls to the rabbinate to interpret and establish the *halacha* in each generation. This has been the nature of rabbinic Judaism since the destruction of the Second Temple in 70 CE.

In order for rabbis to perform this function responsibly, a three-way partnership must exist between physicians and patients, physicians and decisors and patients and decisors. Only in an environment built upon mutual respect, trust and understanding can rabbis effectively serve as facilitators to provide patients and physicians with appropriate religious guidance. Individual patients and doctors must establish links with their own rabbis in order to discuss ethical problems that arise. We are taught in *Ethics of the Fathers* (*Pirkei Avot* 1:16): *"Aseh lecha rav"* (appoint a teacher for yourself) to serve as a mentor and as a partner in one's spiritual, intellectual and moral development. When executed properly, such a relationship is symbiotic, with each party benefiting from the wisdom of the other.

In many instances, rabbis have a difficult task handling problems that are presented to them involving medical ethics. Frequently they do not have the requisite scientific knowledge to comprehend complex medical issues and arrive at a *p'sak* (halachic decision). They must question the physician and the patient carefully and perhaps obtain additional medical information. In many cases, the issues may be beyond their capability and the case referred to a *rav* with more expertise, such as those authorities mentioned earlier (Chapter 2).

Experience over the past few decades has borne out that by establishing and maintaining a system based upon honest and open communication, commitment and trust among all of the parties, Judaism can effectively answer the most difficult dilemmas in the area of medical ethics. Solutions can be reached that are both logical and compassionate, affirming the Jewish tradition's respect for the dignity of the individual.

## Chapter 5: ISSUES IN THE TREATMENT OF ILLNESS

*Devorah is angry about her family's increased incursion into her life and begins to behave rebelliously, plotting to deter them. She creates obstacles to the observance of the Sabbath, when certain categories of "work" are prohibited. For example, Mara shops and prepares meals on Thursday night for* Shabbat. *When her mother's back is turned, Devorah throws the food into the garbage; by the time Mara goes to serve meals on Friday evening, she discovers that the food is gone. The lack of a proper meal creates problems for the entire family since cooking and shopping are prohibited on the Sabbath, but especially for Devorah, since her diet is restricted. On several occasions,*

*Devorah's improper eating has necessitated trips to the emergency room.*

Much of Jewish ritual and heritage is intimately associated with designated periods of sacred time -- embodied in the observance of *Shabbat*. Examining the need to violate the Sabbath in order to preserve life will provide insight into the priority given to life in Jewish tradition.

**Issues:** Sanctity of Life
Violation of the Sabbath to Save a Life

**Sanctity of Life and Violation of the Sabbath to Save a Life**

It is axiomatic in Jewish tradition that life is sacrosanct and of infinite and supreme value. The Talmud (BT, *Sanhedrin* 37a) states: "Therefore, only a single human being was created in the world, to teach that if any person caused a single soul to perish, Scripture regards him as if he had caused an entire world to perish; and if any human being saves a single life in Israel, Scripture regards him as though he had saved an entire world." Therefore, all Biblical prohibitions are suspended in order to save a human life, with the exception of murder, idolatry and prohibited sexual relations (BT, *Yoma* 85a). [For these three "cardinal" sins, the law is that one should allow oneself to be killed rather than transgress.]

Judaism values every moment of life, stringently prohibiting the shortening of life or the hastening of death. The Mishnah (*Semachot* 1:1) states,

> "One who is in a dying condition (*goses* in Hebrew) is considered as a living person in all respects.... One is not permitted to bind his jaws, to stop up his openings, nor place metallic or cooling vessels upon his navel until such time that he dies.... One may not move him, nor place him on sand or salt until he dies. One may not close the eyes of a dying person. He who touches them or moves them is shedding blood because R. Meir used to say: This can be compared to a flickering flame. As soon as one touches it, it becomes extinguished. So, whoever closes the eyes of a dying person is regarded as having taken his soul..."

In another location, the Talmud (BT, *Shabbat* 151b) reiterates this: "He who closes the eyes of a dying person while the soul is departing is like a murderer. This may be compared to a lamp that is going out. If a man places his finger upon it, it is immediately extinguished." Maimonides, in his Mishneh Torah (*Hilchot Avel* 4:5), further expounds:

> "One who is in a dying condition is regarded as a living person in all respects. It is not permitted to bind his jaws, to stop up the organs of the lower extremities, or to place metallic or cooling vessels upon his navel in order to prevent swelling. He is not to be rubbed or washed, nor is sand or salt to be put upon him until he expires. He who touches him is like one who sheds blood. To what may he be compared? To a flickering flame, which is extinguished as soon as one touches it...."

Similar sentiments were later expressed by R. Caro (Sh Ar, *Yoreh Deah* 339).

The importance of life is highlighted by the Talmudic dictum (BT, *Chullin* 10a) of "*hamira sakanta me'issura*" (danger to life and health takes priority over religious restrictions). This principle is amplified by a Talmudic discussion (BT, *Yoma* 85b) concerning the conditions under which it is appropriate to violate the Sabbath.

> "... R. Simeon b. Menassia said: And the children of Israel shall keep the Sabbath. The Torah said: Violate one

> Sabbath so that he may keep many Sabbaths. Rabbi Judah said in the name of Samuel: If I had been there, I should have told them something better than what they said [based on the Biblical verse "You shall study and observe My laws and live by them" (*Leviticus* 18:5), meaning that he shall live by them, but he shall not die because of them."

This is further amplified by R. Natan in the same Talmudic passage: " ...We are told: 'The children of Israel will keep the Sabbath, to observe the Sabbath through the generations' (*Exodus* 31:16). This means, violate one Sabbath in order to observe many Sabbaths afterward."

It is evident, because the discussion about the sanctity of human life occurs in the context of violating the most holy of times, the Sabbath, that this concept is of tremendous importance. The Sabbath, established as an eternal sign commemorating God's role in the creation of the universe, is central to Judaism. Remembering and observing the Sabbath is the only ritual referred to in the Ten Commandments (*Exodus* 20:8-11, *Deuteronomy* 5:12-15). With the exception of Yom Kippur (the Day of Atonement), which occurs annually, *Shabbat* is the most sacred time in Jewish life and under certain circumstances, deliberate desecration of the Sabbath was considered a capital offense.

Almost limitless concerns arise regarding the violation of the Sabbath in order to care for a sick person. These include the types of illnesses in question and whether the laws of *Shabbat* are completely abrogated (*hutra*) or only suspended (*d'chuya*), as well as a host of specific problems relevant to patients and physicians. Although many of these do not constitute ethical dilemmas per se, they have practical implications for physicians and patients, and provide insights into the Jewish tradition's understanding of life and death issues and the halachic process.

*Halacha* recognizes four types of illness. The most serious type is a *choli she'yesh sakana* (an illness that is dangerous), which poses an immediate or potential threat to life, requiring *pikuach nefesh* (the saving of life). A person afflicted with such an illness is called a *choleh she'yesh bo sakana* (sick person for whom there is a danger). The standard employed by *halacha* in determining the risk to life is generally more liberal than that used in current medical practice and may depend upon the perception of the physician, or the patient. Examples of the types of conditions mandating *pikuach nefesh* (Sh Ar, *Orach Chayim* 328:1-16; SSK

32) include internal injuries or wounds, severe pain that could be associated with a serious condition (such as chest pain), infections or abscesses that can progress to a systemic infection, serious internal or external bleeding, conditions associated with a "high" fever, major trauma, fractures, deep lacerations requiring sutures, burns, certain animal or insect bites, loss of consciousness, and poisoning. One is permitted to violate the Sabbath for the sake of a woman giving birth (and for a week after childbirth) and for a fetus that is in danger (SSK 36:2-8). Also, one may violate the Sabbath in the case of emergencies such as natural disasters, fires and falls as a preventative or a therapeutic measure. Persons who are hospitalized are generally considered to be at significant risk and in the category of *choleh she'yesh bo sakana* (a sick person for whom there is a danger) according to R. Feinstein.

The next most serious type of illness is known as *sakanat eyver* (danger to a limb) or *chesron eyver* ([loss of] ability of a limb or organ) (Sh Ar *Orach Chayim* 328:17). Certain injuries affecting the eyes, hands and feet, are specifically delineated by the Talmud as requiring *pikuach nefesh,* while others, such as deep lacerations at risk for infection, can progress to such a point, and are thus treated as such. Examples of conditions in which there is the chance of loss of an organ or limb, or the normal functioning of an organ or limb, but not a threat to life, include minor traumatic injuries to an extremity and certain acute dental problems.

The third type of illness is called a *choli she'ein sakana* (illness that is not dangerous) (Sh Ar. *Orach Chayim* 328:13-33). Here, the patient, referred to as a *choleh she'ein bo sakana* (sick person to whom there is no danger), is not in jeopardy of losing life or limb, but feels badly enough to prefer remaining in bed or is generally weakened. Examples include the flu, gastroenteritis, a bad cold or sore throat, a toothache without concurrent infection and a woman between the eighth and thirtieth day postpartum. The least serious type of illness is referred to as *meychush be'alma* (minor discomfort). It includes such disorders as a headache, mild cold or minor sore throat.

Differentiation between these types of illness is often difficult and subjective. If a physician, nurse or other individual with expertise in the field of medicine is available, his or her opinion should be strongly considered. In cases where doubt exists (*safek pikuach nefesh*), or where there is a disagreement between experts, one should be lenient and err on the side of caution (MT, *Hilchot Shabbat* 2:1, Sh Ar, *Orach Chayim* 328:10, SSK 32-35).

The *halacha* also places considerable weight on the patient's perception of his or her condition, regardless of the opinion of the experts because a person is more sensitive to his or her own needs. This is based upon the verse (*Proverbs* 14:10), "The heart knows its own bitterness" (MB, 328:10).

The guidelines used in treating illnesses on *Shabbat* depend on whether the laws of *Shabbat* are abrogated (*hutra*) or suspended (*d'chuya*). If they are *hutra*, then it is as though *Shabbat* does not exist in reference to this particular issue, and the sick person may be treated as he or she would on any other day, without restrictions. If, on the other hand, they are *d'chuya*, then the laws of *Shabbat* are suspended as necessary to treat the particular life-threatening condition. Most authorities, Maimonides (MT, *Hilchot Shabbat* 2:1), R. Caro (Sh Ar, *Orach Chayim* 328:4) and the Chafetz Chaim (MB, 328:14) agree that the laws are suspended (*d'chuya*) in cases where *pikuach nefesh* is necessary (*pikuach nefesh doche Shabbat*); however, the Rama rules that the laws are abrogated (*hutra*). Most contemporary *poskim*, including R. Feinstein and R. Yosef, concur that one should be lenient in these circumstances. Practically speaking, there is little difference between these interpretations since all authorities concur that the physician should do everything necessary in order to fully treat the condition and that nothing should be deliberately deferred until after *Shabbat* (MT, *Hilchot Shabbat* 2:3).

Also at issue is the question of whether a Jew should preferentially seek treatment from a non-Jewish physician on *Shabbat*. If the laws of *Shabbat* were *hutra*, then this would be unnecessary since a Jewish physician would not be constrained. However, if they were *d'chuya,* then it might be better to be cared for by a non-Jewish physician since it still is considered *Shabbat* and having a non-Jewish physician would avoid violating any restrictions. Here too, in cases where it is necessary to perform the *mitzvah* of *pikuach nefesh,* legally there is no practical difference. Maimonides (MT, *Hilchot Shabbat* 2:3) and Chafetz Chaim (MB 328:37) rule, and most contemporary *poskim* concur, that in cases requiring *pikuach nefesh* the most qualified person available should administer treatment: "When such things have to be done, they should not be left to heathens, minors, slaves, …."

Another effect resulting from the distinction between *hutra* and *d'chuya* relates to the actual method of performing the necessary tasks involved in the treatment, that is, whether a *shinuy* (a modification in the technique or performance of a task that makes it less efficient or more tedious -- for example -- writing with one's non-dominant hand) should be used. If the laws were considered *hutra*, then use of a *shinuy* would be unnecessary, but if they were *d'chuya*, then use of a *shinuy* would reduce the violations from *d'oraita* (Biblically ordained) to *d'rabbanan* (a rabbinic prohibition), which are less severe. In practice, this distinction disappears. In cases involving *pikuach nefesh*, a *shinuy* is not used because the treatment should be dispensed with alacrity and in the most efficient manner, and in less critical conditions, a *shinuy* should only be used if the efficiency of the procedure is not compromised.

Based on these principles, a number of specific issues can be addressed. In situations requiring *pikuach nefesh*, physicians, house officers and medical students may use various electrical devices (such as telephones, pagers, elevators, lights, scopes, electrocardiogram machines, ventilators, etc.); this includes turning them off if it is possible they might be needed again on *Shabbat*. They may carry necessary equipment in public places, write critical pieces of information, prescriptions and orders, draw blood, start an intravenous line, tear tape and suture lacerations. None of these require the use of a *shinuy*, nor should they be postponed until after

*Shabbat*, if that would compromise the care or potentially increase the risk to the patient. Physicians and students may also attend important educational conferences or deliver lectures on *Shabbat,* being careful not to violate any prohibitions or cause others to do so. It is permissible for a physician to drive to the hospital to care for a critically ill patient and also to drive home. Permission to drive home is granted so that the physician will not be dissuaded from responding to such emergencies in the future, based upon the principle known as *hittiru sofan mishum t'chillatan* (the end is permitted for the sake of the beginning). Similarly, although ideally fees should not be charged for services rendered on *Shabbat* and *Yom Tov,* if this will deter Jewish physicians from caring for their patients at these times, then it is allowable (R. Waldenberg).

In less serious situations, *sakanat eyver* or *choli she'ein sakana,* the guidelines for treatment are more restricted (MB, 328:47,54,57; SSK 33:2-22). Under these circumstances, most authorities forbid Jews from directly violating Torah commandments, and at most, permit the violation of rabbinic restrictions. Thus, in order to administer any therapy, it may be necessary for a Jew to utilize a *shinuy* or for the patient to seek help from a non-Jew. Regarding the most minor conditions, *meychush be'alma*, all conventional medical treatments, including the taking of medication such as aspirin (with the exception of certain "home remedies"), are generally forbidden on *Shabbat* (MB, 328:2,3; SSK 34:3-11).[3]

The following situations related to violation of *Shabbat* primarily concern the conduct of patients or non-health care professionals caring for them. One may measure the temperature of a patient who appears ill and desecrate the Sabbath if the temperature is "high" and the patient feels sick (greater than 102°F for an adult, but one should not be strict in this regard). If the suspicion of a serious or a potentially serious problem exists, one may telephone a physician and travel to a hospital. If it will provide valuable psychological comfort to a patient or a woman in labor, it is permissible for a family member to ride in order to accompany a sick person to the hospital. However, the accompanying person may not violate the Sabbath in order to return. On *Shabbat*, one may take medication prescribed for a serious or chronic problem

3. In a private communication, Rabbi Elliot Dorff informs me that "these sources refer to a time when people had to mix the medications with a bowl and pestle, and the crushing of the materials in order to make the medicines is what made them prohibited on the Sabbath. Now that aspirin, etc., come in prepared pills, I fail to see why taking them on the Sabbath should be forbidden."

and people with physical impairments who are unable to ambulate may use a cane, walker or other similar device in public.

It is apparent that the *halacha* has evolved so that priority is given to the preservation of life. Even the remote possibility of serious illness (*safek pikuach nefesh*) is enough to mandate the desecration of *Shabbat* by patients and physicians.

***Four months later.*** *Devorah is experiencing more complications of her diabetes. She has begun manifesting signs of gastroenteropathy (difficulty with digestion and movement of the stomach and intestines, causing pain and constipation), worsening eyesight, peripheral neuropathy (numbness and loss of sensation in her legs) and the onset of renal (kidney) dysfunction. Her doctors believe that this progression could be slowed or even halted if her diabetes were under better, "tighter," control. They discuss the possibility of two experimental treatments: the transfer of pancreatic islet cells (the cells in the pancreas that are responsible for the manufacturing and secretion of insulin into the bloodstream for the digestion of sugar), or an injection of a genetically engineered virus that could produce human insulin. Although, the chances that either of these will be successful is only between 10 and 20 percent, success would lead to dramatic* *improvement in her condition, perhaps even a "cure." Viewing this treatment as a "quick fix," Devorah's attitude becomes a bit more positive.*

The possibility of Devorah achieving a "miracle" cure after suffering with such a long, protracted illness exists. Yet, the chance for success is slim, and the cost high, while the risks, although small, are real.

**Issues**: "Experimental" or newer treatments
Genetic engineering

## "Experimental" or Newer Treatments

All medical procedures and treatments are associated with risks. The choice of the most appropriate treatment for any given patient is dependent upon a risk-benefit analysis, weighing these factors against each other. For treatments whose efficacy is known *(refuah bedukah),* this analysis invariably favors the treatment. Alternatively, for those treatments where the efficacy is unproven or less effective (*refuah she'einah bedukah)*, the risk-benefit ratio may not be as favorable. In these cases, a patient may refuse. However, in such instances, a patient retains the prerogative to subject himself to an increased short-term risk of dying (for example, undergo a radical surgical procedure) in order to potentially achieve a long term cure or return to more normal functioning.

Experimental human treatments, hazardous or otherwise, are also examples of *refuah she'einah bedukah.* Therefore, they are optional, but may be undertaken at a patient's discretion if there is an opportunity for a cure or prolonged survival. Equally important is the understanding that a patient has the right to refuse to submit to such unproven and often potentially dangerous therapy.

Another aspect of human experimentation involves participation in a study or clinical trial, the results of which will not benefit the participants. Examples of this include preliminary human studies ("Phase I " and "Phase II" clinical trials) which evaluate safety and test for dosage of new medications, usually based upon the results of earlier animal studies, and "Phase III" clinical trials, which compare the experimental with an established treatment. The results of Phase I or II trials may not be advantageous to the participants directly, and could potentially expose them to some harm. Their major function is to provide data that will allow more definitive testing (Phase III trials) for therapeutic efficacy to be designed and carried out. Phase III trials may provide benefit to or have deleterious effects on patients, depending upon whether the experimental treatment is effective.

The permissibility of participating in Phase I, II or III studies depends upon the hazards involved, since there is a prohibition against placing oneself in danger (BT, *Shabbat* 32a). If the risks to the participant or the potential side effects of the drug or treatment are minimal, then it is permitted by some (TE XIII, #101; LA, II, p 75; CCAR #17; NARR #152), as "the multitude has trodden upon them" (BT, *Shabbat* 129b). However, if the gamble is great and the potential gain small, such as in Phase I or II trials, then participation is generally prohibited (TE XIII, #101; LA, II, p 75; CCAR #15; NARR #152). Humans do not exert unrestricted proprietorship over their own bodies and may not sacrifice them in order to save another's: "Why do you think his blood is redder than yours" (BT, *Sanhedrin* 74a). But, in cases where there may be a favorable outcome for the patient, and a better alternative does not exist, such as in a Phase III trial or a new antibiotic or anti-cancer drug, then it would be permissible, provided that the patient is fully aware of the hazards involved.

Judaism sanctions animal experiments performed for medical research provided that all appropriate precautions are taken to ensure safety and alleviate pain and suffering (TE XIV, #68; NARR #154). Jewish tradition recognizes a clear hierarchy in the world. Creation occurred in ascending order, from the simplest plants and life forms to the most complex mammals, culminating in mankind that was created *b'tselem Elokhim* (in the image of God). Humans are charged with the task to "....be fruitful and multiply; fill the earth and subdue it, and rule over the fish of the sea, the birds of the sky and every living thing that moves on the earth" (*Genesis* 1:28). Nevertheless, animals are living beings and numerous laws exist governing their treatment. The Torah forbids the killing of a mother with its young (*Leviticus* 12:28). Animals that are threshing may not be muzzled and must be allowed to eat freely (*Deuteronomy* 23:25. BT, *Bava Metzia* 87b, 90a) and a person must feed an animal before himself: "Do not eat before you have fed your beast" (BT, *B'rachot* 40a). One is obligated to lighten the load of an overburdened animal (*Exodus* 13:5) and forbidden from inflicting unnecessary pain on an animal (*Exodus* 23:5, BT, *Bava Metzia* 32a). Domestic animals are required to rest on *Shabbat* (*Exodus* 20:10, 23:12, *Deuteronomy* 5:14) and provisions for their feeding must be made. The Talmud (BT, *Shabbat* 128b) also highlights the importance of protecting animals:

"To relieve an animal of pain or danger is a Biblical law, superseding any rabbinic ordinance [on *Shabbat*]." Furthermore, cruelty to animals, known as *tsar ba'alei chayim*, is expressly forbidden in the Torah (*Deuteronomy* 5:6, 22:6, 22:10, 23:25, 25:4). These injunctions are also designed to protect humans against the callousness that would inevitably result from such insensitive treatment of animals.

In the area of experimental therapy, Jewish law has sought to strike a balance between the probable and the possible, the required and the permitted, and paternity and autonomy, based upon respect for the sanctity of life and modified by the dignity of that life. In the area of animal experimentation, Judaism recognizes a hierarchy while maintaining a degree of respect and compassion for the animal's welfare.

## Genetic Engineering

The field of genetic engineering is an outgrowth of the tremendous advances in molecular biology and human genetics that have occurred over the past two decades. New techniques have facilitated the identification of numerous human genes, defects which predispose one to, or are responsible for, various diseases.

For example, genetic defects have been identified that predispose Ashkenazi Jewish women to breast cancer, certain families to colon cancer, and others to clinical depression, schizophrenia, Alzheimer's disease and numerous other conditions. Other defects are known specifically to cause certain inherited, such as phenylketonuria, Gaucher's or Tay-Sachs disease, sickle cell and other congenital anemias and hemophilia and other clotting disorders. In these latter instances, identification of the specific genetic defect allows for the possibility of replacing the missing or malformed gene product, usually an enzyme or protein or the gene itself, to correct the underlying disorder. At present, it is possible to provide patients with a number of genetically engineered proteins, similar to the provision of insulin for patients with diabetes, to treat various congenital problems. However, these treatments are extremely expensive and must be repeated. Genetic engineering also offers the possibility of creating viruses (termed "vectors") containing genes that code for the defective enzyme or protein that can be injected into a host and incorporated into its cells so that the normal enzyme of protein can be produced within the patient. Attempts are also underway to employ this type of "gene therapy" in the treatment of cancer.

Surprisingly, although a number of ethical issues have been raised concerning the use of such technology, there are few halachic concerns regarding the use of genetic engineering, per se. The major halachic concern that arises is based upon the concept that such types of intervention constitute an affront to the basic Divine plan of creation, which, by definition, should be considered perfect (*derech hateva*). According to Nachmanides [Commentary on the Torah (*Leviticus* 19:19)]:

> "...he who mixes two species alters and challenges the work of creation, implying that God failed to properly generate all of the constituents of the universe, any defect in which He would correct..... Accordingly, man must not mix the species kept apart by God in the process of creation (via Torah statute), and thus confound the order of the world."

Support for this argument is based upon the fact that certain mixtures and interbreeding of animals, seeds, and material for clothing are prohibited (*Leviticus* 19:19; Mishnah, *Kilayim* (Ch. 1-9); BT, *Pesachim* 54b). However, selective breeding of animals and plants has been performed for centuries in order to improve the quality of cattle or agricultural products without rabbinic objection. More recently, genetic engineering of plants and animals, a more efficient method of producing desirable traits, has been done successfully as well.

Most authorities feel that the development and use of newer technologies, such as genetic engineering, to heal human illness is permissible, falling under the rubric of the mandate to "....be fruitful and multiply; fill the earth and subdue it...." (*Genesis* 1:28) (Bleich, Dorff, NARR #154). Use of such methods for the purposes of treating established diseases or preventing disease is mandated by the requirement to "Take heed of yourself, and take care of your life" (*Deuteronomy* 4:9) and "Take exceedingly good care of your lives" (*Deuteronomy* 4:15) and the priority given to *pikuach nefesh.* To the extent that such treatment modalities are new, experimental and pose risk, their use is governed by the concerns expressed in the preceding section ("Experimental" or newer treatments*).* Other ethical concerns involving genetic engineering relate to the acquisition and use of such personal genetic information by various third parties, such as the government, insurance carriers, employers or the military, to affect patient employability and insurability, which are addressed in a separate section (Confidentiality and Truth Telling).

*However, Devorah's parents and grandparents, as Holocaust survivors, are especially skeptical of any "medical research" because of the way the Nazis conducted "experiments" on Jews, Gypsies and other prisoners of war. Just hearing the term "medical research" sends chills up their spines. It brings back horrible memories for them, particularly Devorah's grandfather -- himself a subject of the Nazis. Much consultation with their rabbi and Devorah's physicians is necessary to help everyone make this difficult decision. The fact that Devorah suddenly feels so optimistic about this procedure helps motivate her parents to offer their consent.*

This dilemma highlights the concerns and fears that many people share regarding experimental treatments. The feelings of vulnerability, loss of control and being regarded as subhuman "guinea pigs" to be exploited by the scientific and medical communities for their own purposes lead to a level of distrust that often makes the conduct of human experimentation difficult.

**Issues:** Unethical Conduct of Physicians and Scientists during the Holocaust
Proper Conduct of Human Experiments
Use of Improperly Obtained Scientific Data

**Unethical Conduct of Physicians and Scientists During the Holocaust**

The unparalleled role of physicians in caring for the sick and dying has endowed the field of medicine with an exalted status in society. Ideally, physicians develop a unique trust with their patients based on their shared experiences during the healing process.

Because of the personal nature of illness and the vulnerability of the sick, ethics has always been recognized as a crucial component of the practice or "art" of medicine. Ethical principles governing the roles, responsibilities and relationship between physicians and patients have existed and evolved since antiquity. Although lapses in adherence to these principles have occurred in the past, the ethical violations committed by physicians and scientists during the Third Reich were so egregious that the image of physicians will forever remain tarnished. Doctors and scientists developed and implemented Nazi racial policies, facilitating and promoting the horrors perpetrated during their reign. Therefore it is critical to examine the events and the factors that motivated them to gain insight into the susceptibility of people, even those sworn to protect the weakest, to evil ideas that initially seem logical.

The seeds for such policies were planted in the 19th century, a time of scientific and nationalistic upheaval in Europe. The birth of the field of genetics in the latter part of the century, coupled with intense feelings of nationalism that led to the emergence of independent nation states in Europe, helped spawn the eugenics and social Darwinism movements. The resultant emphasis on "nature over nurture" helped transform anti-Semitism from a religious issue to a scientific and racial one. This transition was the catalyst for enormous social, economic and political consequences. Whereas religious anti-Semitism could theoretically be eliminated through conversion, no escape was possible from racial anti-Semitism.

By the early 20th century, the eugenics or racial hygiene (*rassenhygiene,* as it was known in German) movements became well-accepted within the world scientific and academic communities. In Germany, numerous academic departments, research institutes, professorships and journals were established for the study of racial hygiene. Hitler and the National Socialist Party incorporated these concepts into Nazi ideology. In turn, the medical and scientific worlds embraced National Socialism, as they viewed themselves as partners in the creation of a better, more pure, German *volk* (people).

Physicians joined the Nazi party and the SS in greater numbers than any other profession did.

Subsequent to Hitler's rise to power in 1933, physicians and scientists, often of international repute, played influential roles within the Nazi political machine. In this capacity, many helped formulate and implement the racial policies and laws [Civil Service Law (1933), Sterilization and Castration Laws (1933), Nuremberg Race Laws (1935)] that paved the way for the sterilization and euthanasia ("Aktion T4") programs and, ultimately, the Final Solution. As the war progressed, physicians and scientists also engaged in "research" designed to further both the German war effort and Nazi racial ideology. Experiments promoting the war effort included evaluating methods of survival and rescue through high altitude and salt water trials, freezing, cold water and dry cold exposure and experiments testing newer forms of medical treatment (treatment of battle injuries by sulfanilamide, limb transplantation and coagulants; treatment of chemical burns and injuries due to gas attacks; and treatment of infectious diseases such as hepatitis, malaria, typhus, and yellow fever). Experiments designed to enhance Nazi racial ideology included the infamous twin and dwarf experiments of Josef Mengele; serological experiments; the development of a Jewish skeleton collection; and experiments to develop more efficient techniques for mass sterilization and murder.

The magnitude of the ethical abuses that occurred during the conduct of these human "experiments" on prisoners of war, political prisoners, Jews, Gypsies, homosexuals and other *untermenschen* (inferiors and undesirables) were unprecedented (except perhaps for those perpetrated by the Japanese on POWs during WWII). Among the bioethical principles violated were autonomy, beneficence, nonmaleficence, justice, truth-telling, confidentiality, consent to treatment, refusal of treatment and the sanctity of life. Additional ethical issues involving human experimentation included the primacy of participant safety, the protection of subjects and the proper design of studies.

The record demonstrates that physicians and scientists in Germany involved themselves willingly, and oftentimes enthusiastically, in these ventures. No physician was ever imprisoned, tortured or killed for refusal to participate in these horrors. Organized resistance from within the German medical community was sparse. The individuals involved were representative of the mainstream German medical community. The majority of German physicians and scientists, as well as the academic and scientific communities in

Europe and North America, were well aware of what was occurring in Germany during the 1930s. Regular accounts were published in journals, such as the *Journal of the American Medical Association.* Although the motives varied from ideological to political to financial to personal academic or career advancement, the outcome was the same -- abrogation of those fundamental ethical principles that govern the conduct of physicians and scientists in their relationships to individuals and society.

These atrocities are further magnified by the fact that Germany was one of, if not the most, culturally and scientifically advanced and sophisticated societies in the world at that time, playing a prominent role in medical and scientific research and education. If this could occur in Germany, then why could it not recur elsewhere? Tragically, it does not appear that these actions have been adequately and openly acknowledged by the German (or Japanese) medical communities.

Ethical abuses have also occurred in the United States, including court-sanctioned involuntary sterilization, the Tuskeegee syphilis experiments, the Willowbrook hepatitis vaccine experiments, the Jewish Chronic Disease Hospital experiments and the human radiation experiments, among others. Since these breaches, ethical guidelines for physician behavior and for the conduct of experiments on human beings and the protection of human subjects have been devised.[4]

There are several philosophical issues to consider whenever discussing the Holocaust in an ethical context. One question involves the "uniqueness" of the Holocaust in world and Jewish history and, consequently, whether any extrapolation from the Holocaust to other historical venues is legitimate. Is discussion and analysis of this material appropriate or is it inherently immoral and thus potentially offering legitimization to events that are impossible to justify? These and similar questions continue to plague Holocaust scholars. Therefore, the challenge to those teaching about the Holocaust in related fields such as medical ethics is to universalize certain aspects of the Holocaust experience without trivializing any aspects of it. Utilizing the Holocaust in such a manner does not imply that one can

4. Between 1910 and 1933, nearly 15,000 people in the United States were subjected to involuntary sterilization. In the Tuskeegee (Alabama) syphilis experiments, African-American men with known syphilis were followed for years without treatment to observe the "natural history" of the disease. In the Willowbrook hepatitis vaccine experiments, severely retarded inmates were deliberately injected with live hepatitis B virus in order to test the vaccine. In the Jewish Chronic Disease Hospital case, researchers injected live liver cancer cells into patients to study their immune response. In the human radiation experiments conducted during the Cold War, serious breeches of informed consent policy were identified in subjects given high doses of radiation as treatment for their disease. (Beecher, H.K., "Ethics and Clinical Research." NEJM 274 (1066) 1354-1360)

explain, understand, rationalize, minimize, excuse or condone it. Without attempting to prove moral equivalency, if one wants to use the Holocaust as a successful teaching tool, it must be presented as a part of history -- not apart from history.

**Proper Conduct of Human Experiments**

Awareness of abuses and ethical violations in the conduct of human experimentation over the past few decades has increased efforts aimed at prevention and control. As a result of the Nuremberg Medical Case (United States v. Brandt et al, Subsequent Proceedings, 1946), a number of codes of conduct for experimentation on people and for the protection of human subjects have been developed. Regulations for the ethical conduct of human experiments include the World Health Association's Declaration of Geneva, the American Medical Association's Principles of Medical Ethics and the Constitution of the World Health Organization. Guidelines for the conduct of human experiments include the Nuremberg Code, the American Hospital Association's Patient's Bill of Rights, the World Health Association's Declaration of Helsinki and the U.S. Department of Health, Education and Welfare Regulations on Protection of Human Subjects.[5]

These documents share a number of central elements. For example, proper conduct of these types of experiments requires that they be based upon a reasonable scientific hypothesis, that preliminary work in cells or lower animals support the hypothesis, that additional data cannot be obtained other than from humans, that the experimental end points do not expose the subjects to undue risk and that the experimental design be correct, containing adequate numbers of subjects and controls. Appropriate provisions for the protection of the experimental subjects include: the assurance of free and voluntary, fully informed consent on the part of each subject and that the risks to the subjects be proportional compared to the benefits, the ability of the subject to withdraw from the study at any time without penalty, the exclusion of minors and others unable to properly give consent, the

---

5. The Nuremberg Code {Trials of War Criminals Before the Nuremberg Military Tribunals, 1949]; American Hospital Association: A Patient's Bill of Rights [American Hospital Association House of Delegates, February 6, 1973]; The World Medical Association: Declaration of Helsinki [World Medical Assembly, Helsinki, Finland, 1964, and revised 1975]; Department of Health, Education and Welfare Regulations on the Protection of Human Subjects [Code of Federal Regulations, Title 45, U.S. Code, Part 46, revised January, 1978.]

assurance that adequate pain control is provided and the existence of proper external, impartial monitoring of the study and all procedures.

Within these parameters, Judaism supports the development of newer medical treatments as part of the human mandate to "...fill the earth and subdue it, and rule over the fish of the sea, the birds of the sky and every living thing that moves on the earth" (*Genesis* 1:28). The tradition recognizes the need for scientific investigation involving human subjects; *halacha* provides for participation under the aegis of a *refuah she'einah bedukah.*

## Use of Improperly Obtained Scientific Data

No assurances are foolproof and situations inevitably arise in which it is discovered that scientific data has been tainted by an ethical violation. Such errors may be intentional or unintentional, and may or may not be associated with actual harm occurring to the subjects. Nevertheless, the question of what to do with such data, and whether or not to use, publish or cite it, is serious and can have significant consequences.

Unfortunately, this discussion is often couched in terms of using the data obtained as part of the infamous "Nazi medical experiments." In this instance, except for offending our sensibilities as human beings, there is little practical significance to the question, since virtually all scientific authorities, including the members of the Nuremberg Tribunal itself, have concluded that these so-called experiments were methodologically flawed and produced no useful scientific information. Therefore, it would be more appropriate to consider other examples in which the outcome would have more tangible consequences. For example, consider a case in which an effective treatment for HIV or cancer was discovered. Just prior to publication and dissemination of the results, it became known that there were ethical violations regarding the process of obtaining informed consent. Thus, the decision to withhold the results could adversely affect people's lives by denying them a new treatment until the results could be repeated and properly validated.

Situations such as the one described represent difficult and controversial ethical dilemmas. Arguments are advanced, based upon humane and sentimental considerations, that the results should be published because people's lives are at stake. Perhaps the subjects themselves, whose rights were violated, may desire the disclosure of such findings. Publishing ethically tainted data, however, may reward "eating the forbidden fruit" and promote similar indiscretions in the future. While many may disagree with the idea that such a solution punishes the innocent, it is consistent with the position taken in the American legal system regarding the use of illegally obtained evidence or confessions. In such cases, when the protections afforded to suspects in the areas of self-incrimination and search and seizure are violated, the illegally obtained entities are excluded from evidence, even if it results in a guilty person being freed.

The halachic position articulated by R. Bleich, differs from this. The case against utilizing immorally obtained data is based on two halachic principles. First, there is a prohibition against deriving *hana'ah* (benefit) from the dead; the use of data from subjects who were killed would constitute such a benefit. Second, there is a requirement to dispose of instruments involved in killing together with the victim or perpetrator, implying that the data, as the implement of the crime, must be disposed of because it is tainted. However, several examples are cited which demonstrate that such reasoning does not apply to medical knowledge acquired indirectly through illicit means. There are no rabbinic responsa prohibiting a physician who was forbidden to study medicine (such as a *Kohen*) from practicing once he or she has acquired his or her degree. That is, even though *l'chathilah* (to begin with) it was prohibited for such an individual to study medicine, *b'dieved* (after the fact) it is permissible to utilize this knowledge in order to earn a living and to benefit the sick. Several accounts in the Talmud sanction the use of information gained dishonestly. In order to determine the number of organs in the human body, the students of R. Ishmael boiled and dissected the body of a harlot that had been executed (BT, *B'rachot* 45a). Elsewhere, the Talmud describes the examination of bones inside a synagogue in order to determine whether they were from a single body (BT, *Nazir* 52a). Lastly, the Talmud (BT, *Niddah* 32b) describes a case in which Cleopatra had an abortifacient administered to her female servants and then had them impregnated to study the anatomical differences between male and female fetuses at 40 days of gestation. Even use of this information was permitted.

The halachic position on this issue is that the use of such illegally or immorally obtained information for the purposes of *pikuach nefesh* is permitted: "Everything may be utilized for healing, except for idolatry, sexual licentiousness and homicide" (BT, *Pesachim* 28a). Such a ruling does not preclude the imposition of sanctions or penalties on the perpetrators. It may be appropriate to refuse to give credit to the authors of such a study and to discipline them legally and professionally for their conduct, which might serve as a deterrent against future abuses.

*Devorah's family is finally convinced that it is reasonable to attempt an Islet cell transfer. However, her insurance carrier, a managed care company, refuses to authorize the treatment because it is experimental. The family begins a lengthy appeal process, but to no avail. The company refuses to give in and cover the procedure and she must forego it. Understandably, Devorah is disappointed, yet decides to persevere with the assistance and support of her family.*

It would be nice, simple, if all things in life were equal -- equally pleasant, valuable, available and functional. Unfortunately, they are not. This is especially true in medicine, where such commodities as human organs for transplantation, blood products, specialized equipment and facilities such as intensive care units or operating rooms are often in limited supply in the face of great demand.

The finite supply of precious resources necessitates that choices be made. Such decisions must reflect priorities that have been established based upon a set of previously devised criteria. In

Western societies, these guidelines are based upon the ethical value of distributive justice that incorporates the principles of fairness and the perceived worth of human life.

**Issues:** Triage, rationing and allocation of medical resources

## Triage, Rationing and Allocation of Medical Resources

Assigning responsibility for individual and communal health is a complex task. On an individual level, there are Biblical admonitions to "Take heed of yourself, and take care of your life" (*Deuteronomy* 4:9); "Take exceedingly good care of your lives" (*Deuteronomy* 4:15); "When you shall build a house, you shall make a railing around the roof, that you shall not bring blood upon your house if any man fall from there" (*Deuteronomy* 22:8). The Talmud contains a number of similar pronouncements, such as "A man should not place himself in danger" (BT, *Shabbat* 32a).

While these statements offer general guidelines that promote "healthy" lifestyles, there are also Talmudic prescriptions specifically related to personal health care: "Whoever is in pain, let that person go to the physician" (BT, *Bava Kamma* 46b). In addition, the community's responsibility for providing access to health care is derived from the Talmudic prohibition against a scholar residing in a town without a physician (BT, *Sanhedrin* 17b): "A Torah scholar should not live in a city without: a court..., a charity fund, a synagogue, public bathhouses, toilets, a *mohel* [for ritual circumcision], a physician, a scribe, a butcher, and a teacher [of Torah]...."

Throughout history, Jewish communities have provided these basic types of social welfare services, while balancing individual and communal responsibilities. For example, levels of personal accountability were established as well as methods prioritizing the utilization and disbursement of community resources. These principles are best illustrated by the laws dealing with *tzedakah* (charity) and *pidyon sh'vuyim* (redemption of prisoners), which are performed based upon a set hierarchy.

The laws of *tzedakah* establish two important principles. First, everyone is obligated to give, "even the poor person who is himself sustained by charity must give..." (MT, *Hilchot Matanot L'aniyim* 7:5) and "If a person does not want to give charity... the court may compel him...until he gives as much as the court deems is proper..." (MT, *Hilchot Matanot L'aniyim* 7:10). Second, one's responsibility to those closest to himself exceeds that to those more distant, as it is stated, "...one who gives charity...must prefer them [his family] to others...and the poor of his own household take precedence over the poor of his city, and the poor of his city take precedence over the poor of another city" (Sh Ar, *Yoreh Deah*, 251:3).

The laws of *pidyon sh'vuyim* establish five additional principles. First, each person is responsible for himself, as it is written: "If one is captured and has property, but refuses to redeem himself, then we redeem him [using his resources] against his will." (Sh Ar, *Yoreh Deah* 252:11).

Second, the most vulnerable are given priority in redemption: "We redeem a woman before a man. But, if the captors will engage in sodomy, we redeem the man before the woman."

The third principle establishes equality among people, regardless of social or other considerations: "...if heathens told [a group of Jews]: "Give us one of you to kill or we will kill all of you," then they should all allow themselves to be killed rather than turn over a single soul of Israel [to the heathens]." (MT, *Yesodei HaTorah* 5:5).

Finally, the fourth and fifth principles teach us that there are limits to societal obligations: "We do not redeem captives for more than they are worth....However, an individual may redeem himself for as much as he would like" (Sh Ar, *Yoreh Deah* 252:4). Also, "anyone who does not need charity, yet deceives the community and takes [charity], will not die until he does indeed require charity from others..." (Sh Ar, *Yoreh Deah* 255:2).

These principles, that everyone is equal and obligated to help themselves and others, that those closest and most vulnerable receive priority, and that resources are finite and are not to be abused, provide a sound ethical basis for establishing public policies in this area. For example, the *Shulchan Aruch* (*Yoreh Deah* 249:16) states: "... the obligation to give money for children to study Torah or for the sick and poor takes precedence of the obligation of building and supporting a synagogue."

The overriding attribute governing the implementation of communal policy is justice, which is highly regarded in Jewish tradition. The Torah (*Deuteronomy* 16:20) states: "Justice, justice shall you pursue." Elsewhere, judges are instructed to "judge your neighbor righteously; nor shall you favor a poor man in his cause" (*Leviticus*19:15). With respect to human life, the Talmud prohibits the taking of one life over another: "We do not set aside one life in favor of another" (BT, *Sanhedrin* 72b); and the forfeiting of one life for another, "What makes you think that your blood is redder than his?" (BT, *Pesachim* 25b; *Sanhedrin* 74a).

In the past, European Jewish communities, known as *kehillot*, enjoyed considerable autonomy despite their not being politically independent. They often governed themselves, functioning as self-contained entities within a foreign state, and were largely left alone as long as they paid their necessary taxes. Thus, issues of personal status and civil matters were usually adjudicated according to *halacha* by religious courts. These courts had the authority to tax individuals as they saw fit and establish funds for the public good (Sh Ar, *Choshen Mishpat* 163:1-3). Among the items covered by these funds were defense fortifications, synagogues, *mikvaot* (ritual baths) and salaries for rabbis, teachers and physicians, in order to ensure that these essential services were available to the Jewish community. Thus, although Jewish law does not advocate or promote any particular type of health care delivery system, nationalistic or socialized health care systems are certainly more consistent with those that existed throughout that long segment of Jewish history.

American society's capitalistic system, on the other hand, poses challenges to be addressed by Jewish tradition. In the United States, individuals are more responsible for their own health care and insurance than in nationalized or socialized systems. Is one halachically required to have health insurance in the United States, or is it acceptable to rely on government support in case of illness, even if one can afford insurance? The permissibility of purchasing life insurance has been addressed by R. Feinstein (IM, *Orach Chayim* II #111), who found it acceptable according to *halacha*, comparable to any other prudent business practice and not an expression of doubt in the ability of God to provide for one's needs. In terms of health insurance, one could make the case that it is strongly advisable, if not obligatory, considering the high cost of health care today. Not only do individuals have a duty to care for themselves (*Deuteronomy* 4:9; 15) and to avoid danger (*Deuteronomy* 22:8; BT, *Shabbat* 32a), but they are forbidden to rely unduly on miracles (BT, *Kiddushin* 39b; *Shabbat* 32a) or to rely heavily on others (BT, *Menachot* 103b; Sh Ar, *Yoreh Deah* 255:2). For those individuals that legitimately cannot afford to purchase health insurance, Jewish tradition suggests that it is the community's (i.e., the government's) responsibility to ensure that adequate health care is available to all citizens. Of note, the Talmud (BT, *Avodah Zarah* 55a) declares: "At a time when afflictions are brought upon a person, they are decreed not to depart other than on a specific day, a specified time and at the hands of a specified individual." This statement supports the notion that patients may require the services of certain doctors in his or her treatment, and therefore, must have freedom of choice. This emphasis is contrary to the trend among most current health insurers and managed care corporations to create closed networks of providers, limiting a patient's choice of physician.

Jewish tradition would also suggest other duties incumbent upon the government or its agents, the health insurance industry. While it is true that limits are recognized by *halacha*, the sanctity of life remains paramount. Only in situations that are hopeless or futile are allowances made to forfeit a life or consider cost. For example, in discussing the case of heathens surrounding a town and demanding the release of a Jew, Maimonides (MT, *Yesodei HaTorah* 5:5) rules that "all allow themselves to be killed rather than turn over a single soul of Israel [to the heathens]" unless it is a particular individual that is singled out and that individual is already wanted for a capital offense. In other words, all may not, need not, die if one was already destined to do so. Similarly, the Talmud also establishes priorities in situations where resources are critically limited, such as the famous story in BT, *Bava Metzia* 62a. Two people are crossing the desert and have only enough water for one to survive the trip. Ben Patura argues that they should share the water, even if the result is death for both, so that one would not survive at the expense of the other. R. Akiva disagrees, stating that the owner of the water should keep all of it so that at least he can survive: "Your life comes before that of another." The law goes according to R. Akiva. Financial limitations are also given consideration when redeeming captives: "We do not redeem captives for more than they are worth" (Sh Ar, *Yoreh Deah* 252:4). Here, the purpose of the law is to deter further kidnappings, which would undermine the social fabric of society. Otherwise, it is praiseworthy to redeem prisoners as quickly as possible.

While allocation and rationing of resources is a societal responsibility, the treatment of individual patients is often the individual obligation of a particular physician or health care provider. In terms of an individual physician's role regarding such choices in the treatment of patients, several principles can be elucidated from the halachic sources. First, a person being cared for has priority over someone yet to be treated. This means that a physician is not permitted to abandon a sick patient to administer to another individual at the former's expense, nor can equipment be removed from a patient to treat another if it will result in harm (TE IX 17,10:5; 18:3; NA, *Yoreh Deah* 252:2). In situations where individuals simultaneously require care, attention should be directed at the sicker patient first, provided that his or her chance for survival is reasonable. Alternatively, if the patient that arrived first has almost no chance of survival, the patient with the better prognosis should be seen first (NA, *Yoreh Deah* 252:2; TE XVII 10, 72). In less critical situations, it is appropriate to follow the customary practice in contemporary society whereby all patients are considered equal and treated on a first-come, first-serve basis (IM, *Choshen Mishpat* II #74:1). These halachic guidelines are consistent with those generally in use in the triaging of civilian patients. Conservative (R. Dorff) and Reform (ARR #75) responsa are in agreement with these guidelines for triage.[6]

---

6. It should be noted here that it was Rabbi Elliot Dorff who first used the legal precedents of *tzedakah* and *pidyon sh'vuyim* as a basis for articulating a Jewish position on the distribution of health care. See his *Matters of Life and Death*, c.12.

Triage priorities in military situations are drastically different. In the treatment of civilian populations, where the goal is to care for every patient as well as possible, priority is usually given to the most critically ill patients. In military encounters, where the goal is to return as many fit individuals to the battlefront as quickly as possible, precedence is given to the least injured. Soldiers that are severely injured may be left to die depending upon the number of less injured victims that require treatment. This too is consistent with the halachic parameters for triage outlined above.

In summary, the halachic approach to triage and rationing is based upon the respect and value that Judaism accords each individual, within a broader context of justice and equality.

***Six months later.*** *Devorah requires frequent admissions to the hospital. Her renal failure has progressed and she now needs hemodialysis treatments three times a week. She has become depressed and despondent to the point of being suicidal, and does not want to continue dialysis. Once, when she was home alone, she took an overdose of pills which, while ultimately harmless, demonstrated her intention to end her life and suffering. She is often at odds with her family and health care givers as they insist* *that she continue treatment. She has begun incessantly drinking and smoking cigarettes and even marijuana. These indulgences, which further impair her health, are a chronic source of strife between Devorah and her family. She feels that this is the one small aspect of her life over which she still has some control. A psychiatrist is consulted.*

Serious concerns are raised in this section about one's responsibility to care for himself, even in the face of ongoing despair.

**Issues**: Suicide
- Harmful Behaviors
  - Smoking
  - Alcoholism and use of illicit drugs
- Psychiatric care

**Suicide**

Suicide is equated with murder in Judaism. The Torah states: "Your blood from your (own) person I require" (*Genesis* 9:5), meaning that God will punish one who spills his or her own blood. The Sages have interpreted this to mean that God will punish this offense in the afterlife and that one who commits suicide has no share in the world to come. This view of suicide is rooted in the Jewish concept that people do not have proprietary rights over their own bodies or life; rather, God entrusts this to humans during their stay on earth. In some respects, suicide can be considered more grievous than murder, since this act precludes the possibility of repentance and, in effect, constitutes a denial of divine mastery over the universe. Even in the face of extenuating circumstances, such as pain and terminal illness, suicide is never condoned (IM, *Yoreh Deah* II #174; CARR # 81; Prouser; Dorff)

On rare occasions, Judaism has accepted suicide when committed as an act of martyrdom for the sanctification of God's name (*al kiddush Hashem*). Several examples of such martyrdom are recorded in the Prophets. In *Judges* (16:23-31), the death of Samson is described: "Samson said: 'Let me die with the Philistines.' And he pulled with all his might and caused the house to fall upon the lords and all the people that were there. Those he slew at his death were greater than those he slew during his life." Later, the first accounting of the death of King Saul (*Samuel* 1 31:1-6) is presented. [The second accounting of King Saul's death is discussed in the **Withdrawing and Withholding Treatment** section].

> "The Philistines attacked Israel...and struck down... the sons of Saul. The battle raged around Saul and some of the archers hit him and he was severely wounded. Saul said to his armor bearer: 'Draw your sword and run me through that the uncircumcised may not run me through and make sport of me.' The armor-bearer refused... so Saul took his sword and fell upon it."

The commentators did not condemn Saul for his terminal act of desperation (referred to as an *anous Shaul*). Rather, it was considered an act of martyrdom, which is required by *halacha* over transgression for the three cardinal offenses of murder, idolatry or apostasy and sexual transgressions such as adultery. Saul's suicide out of fear of being captured, tortured and mocked is construed as avoiding idolatry or apostasy, since it would be an affront to God for this to happen to the King of Israel.

The Talmud contains several examples of martyrdom, most notably the deaths of the ten sages by torture at the hands of the Romans for continuing to teach Torah in defiance of a Roman edict. The most famous example of martyrdom in Jewish history involved the mass suicide of the zealots at Masada during the revolt against Rome. Numerous examples occurred during the Crusades, pogroms of the Middle Ages, and later in Europe and during the Holocaust.

The letter of Jewish law treats intentional suicide and its perpetrators harshly. Victims are denied full burial rights, although the mourners are comforted. "For one who has intentionally committed suicide, we do not occupy ourselves with the funeral rites, and we do not mourn nor eulogize him. We do, however, stand in line for him and recite the mourner's prayer [*Kaddish*] and all that is a sign of honor for the living." (MT, *Hilchot Avel* 1:11). This is also the opinion of R. Caro (Sh Ar, *Yoreh Deah* 345). However, in practice, leniency has always been the rule, affording the deceased every benefit of the doubt in order to afford them full burial and mourning rights and spare the family embarrassment. Only cases in which the person was of clear mind and announced his or her plans beforehand are considered intentional suicides. Therefore, in cases of an individual taking his or her own life, efforts are usually made to attribute such a decision to a psychological lapse resulting from extenuating circumstances. Similarly, children who commit suicide are always considered emotionally immature and never held liable. This sympathetic view has persisted in modern times (ARR #89, 90; Siegel; Prouser).

**Harmful Behaviors – Smoking**

Smoking is the single greatest cause of preventable deaths and diseases in the United States. More people die from tobacco-related diseases each year than from alcohol, illicit drugs, homicide, suicide, trauma and AIDS combined, and the link between tobacco use and cancer is incontrovertible. Yet, the question of whether smoking is prohibited by Jewish law is controversial. Opinions of well-respected halachic authorities exist on both sides of the issue.

Beliefs supporting the prohibition of smoking are based on several sources. The Torah offers general admonitions to safeguard ones health: "Take heed of yourself, and take care of your life" (*Deuteronomy* 4:9) and "Take good care of your lives" (*Deuteronomy* 4:15). The Talmud also prohibits irresponsible behavior: "A man should not place himself in danger" (BT, *Shabbat* 32a). Maimonides (MT, *Hilchot Rotzeach* 11:4), R. Caro (Sh Ar, *Choshen Mishpat* 427, *Yoreh Deah* 116, *Orach Chayim* 170:16) and Rama (Sh Ar, *Yoreh Deah* 116:5) all codify the prohibition against endangering oneself, even extending it to situations that are merely potentially harmful. Examples include: the commandment to place a fence around a roof (*Deuteronomy*

22:8) and to cover a well, the prohibition against drinking water left uncovered which might be contaminated by snake venom, drinking river water at night because one might inadvertently imbibe insects, putting money into one's mouth for fear of transmitting an infectious disease, putting one's hand under one's armpit for fear of transmitting leprosy, leaving a knife in fruit, eating unappetizing food which may be rotten, use of dirty pots or dishes, and two people sharing the same drinking cup. Other risky actions that are forbidden are walking under a leaning wall for fear that it could collapse or walking alone at night in case one might encounter robbers. Rationalizations such as "What concern is it to others if I want to place myself in danger?" are expressly dismissed by all authorities.

Additional lines of reasoning have also been employed to support a religious ban on smoking. These include: the negative commandment known as *ba'al tashchit* (Thou shall not destroy, *Deuteronomy* 20:19) anything useful to mankind (MT, *Hilchot Melachim* 6:10) and the prohibition "A man is not permitted to harm himself" (BT, *Bava Kamma* 91b; also MT, *Hilchot Chovel U'mazik* 5:1; Sh Ar, *Choshen Mishpat* 420:31, 571).

Based upon all of the above, in 1976, Chief Sephardic Rabbi of Tel Aviv, Chaim David Halevy, declared that smoking was a violation of *halacha*. This opinion has been supported by R. Waldenberg (TE XV #39, XVII # 21,22, XXI, #14), Dr. Fred Rosner, the United Synagogue of America (Proceedings of Rabbinical Assembly 1983) and the Central Conference of American Rabbis (5753.23). Most recently, several members of the Orthodox Rabbinical Council of America have concluded that smoking is prohibited according to halachah and should be banned in all synagogues, Jewish institutions and homes (Rabbinical Council of America website: www.rabbis.org/publications).

However, not all authorities agree that smoking violates Jewish law, although they vigorously condemn the habit and strongly discourage people from starting. Although people have been smoking for centuries, its adverse effects on health have only recently been appreciated. Worldwide, there has been no decrease in the incidence of smoking, and the number of women that smoke continues to increase. The concern is purely legal as to whether a ban on smoking can be supported by *halacha.* Feinstein wrote in a 1964 responsum (IM, *Yoreh Deah* II #49):

> "One should certainly take care not to start smoking, and to take proper care in desisting. But, should one conclude that it is forbidden as an activity dangerous to one's health? The answer is that because the multitude are accustomed to smoking and the *Gemara* in such a case invokes the principle of *shomer pta'im Hashem* ('The Lord preserves the simple,' *Psalms* 116:6), tractates *Shabbat* 129b and *Niddah* 31a, and in particular since the greatest Torah scholars in the present and previous generations do or did smoke [it is not forbidden]."

That is, since the majority of people who smoke, even though it may be foolish and unwise, are unharmed and since the risk has generally been accepted by society, then it cannot be considered to violate *halacha*, per se. Rabbis Auerbach (NA, *Yoreh Deah* 511:1, *Choshen Mishpat* 155:2), Yosef, and Bleich support this view.

In addition, Bleich, based upon Rabbi Jacob Ettlinger, notes the difference between an immediate danger and a potential danger. For example, taking a sea voyage or plane ride or having a woman become pregnant does not pose a danger under the majority of circumstances, although there are crashes or disasters which occur. Similarly, cigarette smoking does not pose an immediate danger to most people, but rather constitutes a "potential" risk to the individual that will likely not be realized in the majority of cases.

Lastly, the Talmud states that "we must not impose a restrictive decree (*takanah*) upon the community unless the majority of the community will be able to endure it" (BT, *Bava Kamma* 79b); and "It is better that they should transgress inadvertently rather than be deliberate sinners" (BT, *Shabbat* 148b). Based upon these principles, many leading rabbinic authorities have refused to ban smoking. However, proponents of a halachic admonition against smoking object to this reasoning, saying that these principles should not apply in a case demanding *pikuach nefesh* (saving of a life), in which the risks are supported by strong scientific evidence.

While smoking has not been uniformly forbidden according to *halacha*, exposing bystanders to "second-hand smoke" may present a clearer violation of it. The Biblical phrase, "When you shall build a house, you shall make a railing around the roof, that you shall not bring blood upon your house if any man fall from there" (*Deuteronomy* 22:8), suggests that one has a responsibility to protect other individuals from danger. Similarly, in Talmudic times the Rabbis recognized the hazards of pollution, requiring that "smokestack[s].... be removed from the city...." (Tosefta, *Bava Batra* 1:7). Based on this ruling, it would not be permitted for someone to smoke if a bystander objects (TE XV #39; IM, *Choshen Mishpat* II #18).

The resolution of the halachic problems associated with smoking illustrates some of the concerns faced by *poskim* about the broader implications of their decisions. Although all authorities are opposed to smoking, some do not believe halachic justification exists, or they think that the halachic ramifications of a rabbinic ban on smoking would create more problems than it would solve. Others feel that smoking poses a significant enough threat to life and health that it justifies strong actions. Similar tensions exist in all legal systems.

**Harmful Behaviors – Alcohol and Illicit Drugs**

The benefits and dangers of alcohol and drugs have been recognized since Talmudic times. Alcohol, particularly wine, has played a prominent role in Jewish ritual. Although usually recommended in moderation, such as for the *Kiddush* (ritual sanctification of *Shabbat* or holidays), there are several instances in which drinking is encouraged. Among these is the holiday of Purim, where one traditionally drinks until he cannot tell the "wicked Haman from the blessed Mordechai" and on Passover, when one is required to consume four cups of wine. Various statements endorsing drinking also appear: "Wine gladdens man's heart" (*Psalms* 104:15), "Now that the Temple is no longer in existence, there is no rejoicing except with wine" (BT, *Pesachim* 109a), and "All who are sated with wine have the characteristics of seventy elders" (BT, *Eruvin* 65a). Similarly, the use of drugs for the purposes of restoring health is amply documented in the Talmud and Codes of Law. The Talmud (BT, *Sanhedrin* 43a) even records the fact that convicted criminals were given a potion prior to execution to alter their senses to ensure a comfortable death (an example of the commitment to *k'vod habriut* -- respect for all living beings).

Numerous references to the harmful effects of alcohol are also recorded. The Torah relates the instances of sexual licentiousness associated with the drunkenness of Noah (*Genesis* 9:20-23) and Lot (*Genesis* 19:30-38). The deaths of Aaron's sons for bringing an unauthorized sacrifice in the Tabernacle have been attributed by some to their being under the influence of alcohol: "Drink no wine or ale, you or your sons, with you, when you enter the tent of the meeting, that you may not die. It is a law for all time throughout your generations, for you must distinguish between the sacred and the profane, and between the unclean and the clean" (*Leviticus* 10:9-10). The *Midrash Rabbah* (*Numbers* 10:3) says: "Where there is wine there is immorality." Other scriptural exhortations against drunkenness include: "Wine is a scoffer, strong drink makes one cry out. He who is muddled by them will not grow wise" (*Proverbs* 20:1) and "Do not be those who guzzle wine or glut themselves on meat; for guzzlers and gluttons will be poor...." (*Proverbs* 23:20-21).

The Talmud highlights the negative characteristics of alcohol (wine) and its effects on intellectual functioning. "As wine enters, secrets leave" (BT, *Sanhedrin* 38a) and "For nothing else but wine brings woe to man" (BT, *Sanhedrin* 70b). "He who loves wine and oil does not grow rich" (*Proverbs* 21:17). Wine has also been linked to misery, poverty, rage, confusion, and perversion of justice (*Proverbs* 20:1; 21:17; 23:19-21, 29-35; 31:4,5). The psychological and cognitive effects of alcoholism are also addressed in the rabbinic prohibitions involved in performing *mitzvot* while under the influence of alcohol. This is codified by Maimonides (MT, *Hilchot Tefillah* 4:17):

> "One who is drunk should not pray; but if he does his prayer is an abomination. One who has imbibed should not pray; but if he does, his prayer is a prayer. What is the definition of drunk? One who cannot speak coherently in the presence of a king. One who has imbibed is able to speak before a king without becoming confused."

It is also forbidden for a man who is drunk to request a *get* (decree of divorce) or to appear in court even after a small amount to drink. Thus, it is apparent that while Jewish tradition accepts a role for wine and alcohol, skepticism and warnings about the dangers of excess prevail.

The Sages acknowledged the potential adverse effects of repeated drug use. The possibility of side effects was noted in the statement: "When a man gives a drug to his fellow, it may benefit one limb, while injuring another..." (BT, *Eruvin* 54a). Elsewhere in the Talmud (BT, *Pesachim* 113a), Rav admonishes his son: "Do not take drugs." Rashbam, in commenting on this statement, writes: "Do not drink drugs because they demand periodic doses and your heart will crave them. You will waste much money thereby. Even for medical care, do not drink them, and if possible find another mode of healing" (see also Maimonides, *Commentary on the Mishnah*, *Bava Kamma* 90a). This suggests that there was an appreciation in Talmudic times of the potential for addiction. In contemporary society, considerable attention has been focused on the adverse effects of alcohol and illicit drugs. The use of alcohol and drugs continues to increase in American teens, despite the availability of drug and alcohol prevention programs. Teenagers and young adults, who constitute about 20 percent of all licensed drivers, account for 40 percent of all vehicular accidents. The health toll related to alcohol and drugs, although less than smoking, is enormous. Nevertheless, the halachic positions taken regarding their use are controversial.

In terms of drinking, there has been no movement to issue a halachic ban. While major rabbinic authorities deride the dangers of chronic alcoholism and overindulgence, the place of alcohol in Jewish tradition and ritual seems secure. The sight of yeshiva students getting drunk openly on *Purim* or *Simchat Torah* is commonplace as is the sneaking of alcohol at *Shabbatonim* (retreats over *Shabbat*) and teen retreats. Underage drinking frequently occurs despite its prohibition in secular law (*dina d'malchuta dina).*

Rabbinic authorities have been more forthcoming regarding the use of drugs. This is due to several facts: The use of illicit drugs is outlawed in most jurisdictions (*dina d'malchuta dina*), drug use -- unlike smoking and drinking – is less tolerated among society at large, there is greater fear about the hazardous consequences of illegal drug use than of smoking and drinking, and the Jewish tradition is concerned about the dangers of excessive indulgence. Rabbi Feinstein, in a 1973 responsum (IM, *Yoreh Deah* III #35), prohibited smoking marijuana (and presumably all other drugs) for several reasons. Many people taking drugs suffer cognitive deficits, which may impair health and the ability to perform other *mitzvot*, such as prayer or Torah study. Marijuana use may lead to addiction or craving for other drugs, which could result in violence in order to obtain more drugs. Drug usage could precipitate conflict between parents and children, violating the precept to "honor your father and mother" (*Exodus* 20:12). Lastly, use of drugs violates the Biblical prescription to "be holy" (*Leviticus* 19:2). This prohibition against the use of drugs for pleasure is supported by the Reform movement as well (CCAR #73). The Conservative movement has ruled against the use of drugs for pleasure (for example, in United Synagogue Youth policy [which also prohibits underage drinking during its events]) and Rabbi Elliot Dorff has addressed this in *Matters of Life and Death*, p.251.

In contrast to smoking, all rabbinic authorities have taken a negative view of the use of illicit drugs, including marijuana, for the reasons cited. Because of alcohol's "sacred" role in Jewish ritual, however, dealing with its abuse has been more of a problem.

## Psychiatric Care

Contemporary society no longer stigmatizes patients for seeking treatment for psychiatric disorders, such as receiving counseling and medication. Judaism, too, recognizes the importance of mental health and a sense of personal well-being and views such treatment as appropriate when necessary. This opinion is consistent with the general admonitions to "take heed of yourself, and take care of your life" (*Deuteronomy* 4:9) and "take exceedingly good care of your lives" (*Deuteronomy* 4:15). Psychiatric illnesses, such as acute psychosis or severe depression, are accorded the same standing in *halacha* as physiological illnesses, and are classified in the same manner with regard to violation of *Shabbat* and other prohibitions in matters requiring *pikuach nefesh*.

The sages of the Talmud recognized the power of the psychological state and its potential effect on the individual as illustrated by two vignettes. Choni the Circle-Drawer slept for 70 years. After he awoke and identified himself to the people, no one recognized him or believed him, despite his great mastery of Torah. Because of his depression and the feeling that he was "lost" in his new world, he prayed to God for death. His wish was granted (BT, *Ta'anit* 23). The other story stems from the *Midrash*. An elderly woman approached R. Yose ben Chalifa and told him that she was too old, her life no longer had meaning and she wished to die. R. Yose inquired of her how she lived to such an old age, to which she replied that she went to synagogue each morning. He advised her to skip three consecutive mornings. She did as the rabbi suggested and died on the third day. The sages, by verifying the seriousness accorded to the psychological state, condemned neither of these individuals.

Modern *poskim* have similarly acknowledged the importance of psychological and emotional factors in their decisions. R.

Feinstein has granted permission for a loved one to accompany a woman in labor to the hospital on *Shabbat*, and has permitted the use of contraceptives by women who have experienced post-partum depression or have been guilty of child abuse.

The guidelines used in the selection of an appropriate physician or counselor, according to R. Feinstein (IM,*Yoreh Deah* II #57), are similar to those employed for physical disorders: choose the most qualified practitioner. One caveat applies: one is prohibited from being treated by anyone that is engaged in proselytizing or trying to lead one astray from Judaism (BT, *Avodah Zarah* 27b). Fortunately, this is rarely an issue, as most professionals conduct themselves appropriately and do not actively attempt to lure clients away from their religion.

The consideration of an individual's psychological state by halachic decisors along with the recognition of the importance of properly managed psychiatric problems confirms Judaism's appreciation of the unity and interdependence of the human mind and body.

***Eight months later.*** *Because the long-term survival of diabetics on dialysis is poor, doctors recommend that Devorah* *undergo a kidney transplant, which would offer her a better chance for survival and potentially, a more "normal" lifestyle. Living related donors are preferable because their organs offer a greater chance of long- term success. As Devorah's only living blood relative, Rafi, a minor, is the only potential organ donor available. He, however, is afraid of doctors and hospitals, and has expressed doubts about the potential risks posed to him.*

*Rafi's attitude places Mara and Chaim in an untenable position. Do they encourage one child to potentially endanger his health in order to save the life of his sister? They are angry and resentful that they are confronted with these impossible decisions. Rafi cannot help but feel guilty that he is not stepping forward more eagerly to assist his older sister. But, having watched her suffer in the past, he does not want to find himself in a similar position later in life.*

The availability of new, potentially dangerous medical technologies and procedures pose challenging ethical dilemmas for patients and practitioners. The field of organ transplantation is one of the most exciting and rapidly changing in all of medicine. Despite its enormous therapeutic potential, these types of procedures raise a number of halachic issues that are unique to Judaism.

**Issues**: Permissibility and obligation of accepting an organ from a living related donor
Permissibility and obligation for living related organ donation

**Permissibility of Organ Transplantation**

Several halachic issues arise when considering organ transplantation. Primary among these is the permissibility of organ transplantation, evaluated from the perspective of organ reception as well as organ donation.

Since the first kidney transplant was performed in the 1950s, which employed an organ that was harvested from a living relative (living-related transplant), the field of transplantation has progressed remarkably. At this time, transplantation of kidneys (from living-related and from cadaver donors), heart, lung, liver, combined heart-lung, combined kidney-pancreas, bone marrow and corneas are safe and successful. All of these are considered to be conventional treatments and are performed routinely in many medical centers. Transplantation of the small intestine or multiple abdominal organs simultaneously is still considered experimental.

To the extent that these different procedures are part of the normal medical armamentarium, they are halachically acceptable. Furthermore, any patient with a condition requiring a transplant would be considered a *choleh she'yesh bo sakana*, requiring *pikuach nefesh*. Whether acceptance of a transplant is required by *halacha* would depend upon the risk and success of each particular type of transplant (whether each was a *refuah bedukah* or a *refuah she'einah bedukah*). For example, the long-term benefits of kidney, heart, liver and cornea transplants exceed those of lung, bone marrow and combined organ procedures. While rabbinic opinions vary regarding whether any, some or all of these treatments would be obligatory, all would agree that they are permissible.

A patient in danger may risk decreasing short-term life (*chaye sha'ah*) for the possibility of a long-term gain (*chaye olam*), "[When there is a chance for cure] we do not place much value on the final hours of life" (BT, *Avodah Zarah* 27b). The Talmud (BT, *Yoma* 85a) discusses the case of rescuing a person buried under a collapsed building on *Shabbat*. In this instance, the laws of *Shabbat* are set aside (*d'chuya*) in order to attempt to rescue the individual (*pikuach nefesh doche Shabbat*), even if the possibility that he is alive is remote and regardless of how long he may live. The ban against a Jew confronting a life-and-death situation being treated by a heathen who is suspected of malicious motives is also set aside for the remote possibility that the heathen may recant and provide the appropriate care (BT, *Avodah Zarah* 27b). Preference is given to long-term over short-term survival, as evident from the famous Talmudic discussion (BT, *Bava Metzia* 62a) concerning two people crossing the desert who have only enough water for one to survive the trip. R. Akiva advocates that the person owning the water keep it so that at least he can survive, rather than sharing it so that they both die: "Your life comes before that of another."

Authorities differ regarding the degree of success required in order to justify a procedure that may in fact shorten a life. Some require a standard of 50 percent success, while others maintain that short-term survival is of little importance and one may undergo a dangerous treatment even if the chance of success is small. This is illustrated in an early responsum by R. Feinstein (IM, *Yoreh Deah* II #174), stating that heart transplantation was forbidden because the procedure had not been perfected and the risk of death too great. At a later date after survival rates improved (as quoted by R.

Tendler), Rabbi Feinstein modified his position and permitted heart transplantation.

While it is permissible to accept an organ for transplantation, other dilemmas remain. For example, is a Jew permitted to accept an organ from a non-Jew? A related question often raised is whether a Jew may accept tissues (such as a heart valve) or extracts (such as insulin) from non-kosher animals. The answer to both of these questions is that the status of the donor is of no consequence because this is considered an act of *pikuach nefesh*. Furthermore, with respect to the use of animal products, the laws of kashrut only apply to eating, and would be suspended in any case in matters of life or death.

What about the status of a transplant recipient? A *Kohen* (priest) is normally prohibited from having contact with the dead. This restriction is also waived in a life-threatening situation, allowing a cadaver organ transplantation. The individual would also not forfeit his ritual obligations (being called to the Torah as a *Kohen*, administering the priestly blessing, etc.) as a result of having undergone such a transplant.

A number of ethical quandaries regarding organ donation also arise from both living-related and cadaver organ donation. The issues pertaining to living-related organ donation primarily involve risk to the donor. As noted earlier, it is forbidden to sacrifice one's life in order to save another ["Your life comes before that of another" (BT, *Bava Metzia* 62a)] and to deliberately endanger oneself ["Take heed of yourself, and take care of your life" (*Deuteronomy* 4:9). Other sources are: "Take good care of your lives" (*Deuteronomy* 4:15), and "A man should not place himself in danger" (BT, *Shabbat* 32a)]. However, not all risks are equivalent. Certain risks are an inherent part of life ["The multitude has trodden upon them" (BT, *Shabbat* 129b)]. Yet, in Judaism, people are considered to be responsible for one another ["All of Israel is responsible one for the other" (BT, *Shevuot* 39a)] and are legally held to such a standard ["Whence do we know that if a man sees his neighbor drowning or mauled by beasts or attacked by robbers, that he is bound to save him? From the verse 'Neither shall you stand idly by the blood of thy fellow'" (BT, *Sanhedrin* 73a). "Whoever is able to save another and does not save him transgresses the negative commandment, 'Neither shall you stand idly by the blood of thy fellow'" (MT, *Hilchot Rotzeach* 1:14)]. Thus, the issue becomes one of degree. How much risk is one required to assume in order to "save the life of another" without "stand[ing] idly by the blood of one's brother" (*Leviticus* 19:16).

The rabbis have taught that while it is not obligatory to risk one's life to save another, it may be praiseworthy to do so under certain circumstances (Radbaz). He refers to such an individual as *hasid shoteh* (pious fool). According to the *Aruch HaShulchan Choshen Mishpat* 426:4), "...[it] depends on the circumstances. One must weigh the matter on a scale, and not safeguard himself more than necessary." Therefore, the permissibility for one to donate an organ is dependent on the risk of the particular procedure in question. For example, donating blood is permitted, if not mandated, because the dangers and pain involved are minimal (IM, *Choshen Mishpat* #103; NA, *Yoreh Deah* 349,3:3:3). Donation of bone marrow is slightly more hazardous, but only minimally so; however, it is associated with considerably more discomfort. Thus, donating bone marrow is permitted, and some authorities might even consider it to be obligatory (NA, *Yoreh Deah* 349, 3:3:2, *Choshen Mishpat* 420:1). Giving a kidney, on the other hand, entails major surgery. Although still safe (the risk of dying about one per 1,000 donors), it is considerably more dangerous and painful than bone marrow or blood donation. Serving as a living-related donor, although praiseworthy, is optional according to *halacha*, and only if the risk to the donor is minimal (TE IX, #45; NA, *Yoreh Deah* 157, 4:2; ARR #86).

This issue has been addressed in numerous court cases in the United States and Israel. One illustrative Israeli case involved a young, developmentally disabled boy who was being cared for by his father. The child was completely dependent upon the father for his daily living and maintenance. The father became ill with chronic renal disease, requiring dialysis. A question arose as to whether the young man should be compelled to donate a kidney to his father because such a transplant would give the father the best chance for leading a normal life -- which in turn would benefit the son. The Israeli courts decided that the son's right to privacy and bodily integrity outweighed the "best interest" standard and refused to force the boy to donate the kidney. Similar case law exists in the United States. R. Bleich has analyzed this case from a halachic perspective and reached the same conclusion.

The manner in which *halacha* deals with the numerous ethical issues involved in organ transplantation underscores

Judaism's commitment to the sanctity of life and its respect for individual autonomy.

*After observing his sister suffer and deteriorate over time, Rafi eventually consents to becoming an organ donor. However, the medical team reconsiders and feels that a combined pancreas-kidney transplant might be a better long-term treatment option because it could possibly "cure" her diabetes and stop the progression of her complications. Devorah and her family agree for her to undergo a combined pancreas-kidney transplant. Rafi's soul searching and meritorious gesture become moot because a pancreas cannot be taken from a living donor. She is placed on the waiting list for a cadaver transplant.*

***Four months transpire.*** *A serious motor vehicle accident occurs. The victim is a 34-year-old Jewish male, Natan. He has suffered a severe head injury due to blunt trauma along with a lung contusion and pelvic fracture. His condition is critical and after he is initially stabilized in the emergency department, he is transferred to the intensive care unit (ICU) for further care. His condition worsens over the next 48 hours and his physicians believe that his head injury will be fatal. They inform his family,* *initiate an evaluation for neurological or brain death, and notify the organ procurement network and transplant team. The next morning, Natan is pronounced "dead, based upon neurological criteria," and his family is approached about the possibility of organ donation. Although Natan checked off the organ donor box on his driver's license, his family's consent is still required. They quickly consult their rabbi about this difficult decision.*

The psychological travail experienced by the family of a potential organ donor is tremendous. Faced with the shock of having a family member, usually a child, declared brain dead coupled with the request to donate organs is an overwhelmingly emotional ordeal. For Jews, this is further complicated by halachic issues revolving around the definition of death in Jewish law and the permissibility of cadaver organ donation.

**Issues**: Definition of death
Permissibility and obligation for cadaver organ donation

## Definition of Death in Jewish Law

Cadaver organ transplantation requires the removal of the donor organs while a beating heart still perfuses them with blood and oxygen. In order for medical authorities to accomplish this, the classical definition of death, consisting of the irreversible cessation of circulation and respiration, had to be altered. In 1981, the Uniform Determination of Death Act redefined death as: (a) the irreversible cessation of circulatory and respiratory function, or (b) the irreversible cessation of all functions of the entire brain, including the brain stem. Such individuals are colloquially referred to as "brain dead" or "dead by neurological criteria." (This definition does *not* include conditions such as traumatic coma or a persistent vegetative state. Such patients are considered to be alive according to civil law). The dual definition has since been accepted by authorities in all 50 states and virtually around the world.

The Jewish concerns center around the question of whether these medical and legal definitions of death are compatible with the understanding of death as delineated by *halacha*. This remains a controversial and contentious point.

The classic halachic definition of death is the cessation of respiration. It is based upon several Biblical and Talmudic sources: "The Lord formed man of the dust of the ground, and breathed into his nostrils the breath of life, and man became a living soul" (*Genesis* 2:7); and "in whose nostrils was the breath of the spirit of life...died" (*Genesis* 7:22). The Talmud (BT, *Yoma* 85a) expounds upon this issue in the context of a discussion of those circumstances under which the Sabbath may be desecrated:

> Mishnah: "...every danger to human life suspends (the laws of the) Sabbath. If debris (from a collapsed building) falls on someone and it is doubtful whether he is alive or dead, or whether an Israelite or a heathen, one must probe the heap of the debris for his sake (even on the Sabbath). If one finds him alive, one should remove the debris but if he is dead, one leaves him there (until after the Sabbath)."
>
> Gemara: "How far does one search (to ascertain whether he is dead)? Until (one reaches) his nose. Some say: Up to his heart.... life manifests itself primarily through the nose, as it is written: "in whose nostrils was the breath of the spirit of life" (*Genesis* 7:22)...."

Maimonides later codifies the explanation as follows: "If, upon examination, no sign of breathing can be detected at the nose, the victim must be left where he is (until after the Sabbath) because he is already dead" (MT, *Hilchot Shabbat* 2:19). Similarly, R. Caro (Sh Ar, *Orach Chayim* 329:4) writes: "Even if the victim was found so severely injured that he cannot live for more than a short while, one must probe until one reaches his nose. If one cannot detect signs of respiration at the nose, then he is certainly dead whether the head was uncovered first or whether the feet were uncovered first."

However, alternative classical opinions are put forth regarding the halachic understanding of death that requires the cessation of both cardiac and respiratory activity. In commenting on the case of a woman who dies during childbirth where an emergency Cesarean section is performed because the possibility exists that the fetus is still viable (Sh Ar, *Orach Chayim* 330:5), Rama suggests that this practice should no longer be done because of the impossibility of discerning the exact moment of maternal death. The concern is that the patient may have fainted and only appeared dead. The 19$^{th}$-century sage, the Chatam Sofer, ruled that a person could only be declared dead if he had no respiration, no pulse (heartbeat), and the appearance of a "stone" (*rigor mortis*), and suggested that one wait for a period of time before making that decision.

Advocates of the position that total brain death is compatible with *halacha* have employed two lines of reasoning in support of this argument: (1) Modern science dictates that respiratory death implies total brain death, and (2) The analogy is that brain death is similar to physiologic decapitation.

The first explanation, supported by Dr. A.S. Steinberg and R. Auerbach (Assia 1994), states that the halachic guideline for the determination of death is total and irreversible stoppage of spontaneous respiration. The two prerequisite conditions for the determination of death are that the patient appears dead and confirmation that there is irreversible cessation of respiration (the sign of death). When it is clear that these conditions are met, a person is considered dead according to *halacha*. Irreversible cessation of respiration can be verified in one of two ways: irreversible cessation of cardiac activity (which will soon result in total brain death due to anoxia) or irreversible activity of the entire brain (including the brainstem, which completely controls respiration). In either of these circumstances, the halachic definition of death (total irreversible cessation of spontaneous respiration) is achieved.

The second view, advanced by R. Tendler, the Rabbinical Council of America, and R. Feinstein (IM, *Yoreh Deah* II #174, III #132), considers brain death analogous to physiologic decapitation. The Talmud, when discussing ritual impurity (Mishnah, *Ohalot* 1:6), states that an animal that is decapitated is considered ritually impure or unclean (and can transmit ritual impurity) because it is considered dead, regardless of whether it exhibits purposeless motion or twitches after the head has been severed.

> "Absent heartbeat or pulse was not considered a significant factor in ascertaining death in any early religious source. Furthermore, the scientific fact that cellular death does not occur at the same time as the death of the human being is well recognized in the earliest Biblical sources. The twitching of a lizard's amputated tail or the death throws of a decapitated man were never considered residual life but simply a manifestation of cellular life that continued after death of the entire organism had occurred. In the situation of decapitation, death can be defined or determined by the decapitated state itself as recognized in the Talmud and Codes.

Complete destruction of the brain, which includes loss of all integrative, regulatory, and other functions of the brain, can be considered physiologic decapitation, and thus a determinant per se of death. Loss of the ability to breathe spontaneously is a crucial criterion for determining whether complete destruction of the brain has occurred. Earliest Biblical sources recognized the ability to breathe independently as a prime index of life....destruction of the entire brain or brain death, and only that, is consonant with Biblical pronouncements on what constitutes an acceptable definition of death, i.e., a patient who has all the appearances of lifelessness and who is no longer breathing spontaneously. Patients with irreversible total destruction of the brain fulfill this definition even if heart action and circulation are artificially maintained." (JAMA 1977;238:1651-55).

This reasoning implies that Judaism accepts the idea, and has always accepted the notion, that biological death is a continuous process. Various cells and organs die or cease to function at different times, depending upon their relative sensitivity to lack of oxygen, blood or other vital components. Determination of death does not require that signs of decay be present, indicating death of all of the body's cells and organs. Rather, in Judaism, death is determined to have occurred at an earlier juncture that corresponds to the irreversible cessation of respiration, the most reliable sign of death (because it, in fact, signifies that the brain has died).

Thus, if it can be decided that all brain activities, including brain stem functions, have stopped, the patient can be considered dead according to Jewish law. This can be determined by a combination of clinical exams and confirmatory tests (an EEG alone is not acceptable for this purpose). This position was supported by R. Feinstein (IM, *Yoreh Deah* II #174, III #132).

A letter from R. Tendler to Hadassah Medical Center (1986) stated:

> "Heart transplants today have converted from the experimental to the therapeutic category. The halachah, mindful of two critical changes in the surgical protocol, views heart transplants as currently practiced favorably. The changes are: 1) The donor must be brain dead. That is, there must be positive cessation of all brain function, including that of the brain stem. Such a donor is not

> clearly ethically or halachically alive, provided that brain death can be confirmed beyond a shadow of a doubt. We recommend that the best indicator of brain death is the finding of non-circulation of blood in the brain... 2) Though there are clear risks, the surgical benefits for the recipient are overwhelming. My late father-in-law, R. Moshe Feinstein, was well aware of these developments and permitted heart transplants in the later years. Similarly, a neighbor of mine who received a heart-lung transplant two years ago at Dr. Starzl's Pittsburgh center had been advised accordingly by both R. Feinstein and the Lubavitcher Rebbe."

Similarly, in 1987, the Chief Rabbinate of Israel, under direction of the Ministry of Health, investigated this issue and issued a directive which endorsed the notion of brain death as halachic death, while precisely stipulating the circumstances and conditions necessary to proceed with heart transplants in Israel. These conditions are clearly applicable to determining death for other forms of transplantation as well. Both the Conservative and Reform movements have accepted the medical neurological criteria for death as compatible with the halachic definition (R. D. Goldfarb, 1976; R. S. Siegel, 1976; CARR #78).

Opponents of this position (R. Bleich, R. Waldenberg, R. I. Unterman, R. A. Soloveitchik) insist that cessation of cardiac function is also a criterion of death according to *halacha*. Therefore, a patient without neurological functioning is alive as long as there is cardiac activity. Moreover, discontinuance of mechanical ventilation from such a patient is considered murder.

The debate among *poskim* about the precise halachic definition of death exemplifies the struggle and commitment necessary to integrate Judaism and modern society. Yet, this debate also symbolizes the challenges necessary to remain true to the tenets of the Torah in a rapidly changing world.

**Permissibility and Obligation for Cadaver Organ Donation**

Cadaver organ donation is complicated halachically, with the central legal debate revolving around the definition of death. As noted above, if one accepts the argument that total brain death constitutes death according to Jewish law, then the obligation to save a life (*pikuach nefesh*) must be balanced against the principle of *kavod ha'met* (respect for the dead). Respect for the dead entails swift burial, not mutilating the body nor deriving benefit from the dead (*assur b'hana'ah*). Cadaver organ donation potentially compromises each of these aspects.

Burial arrangements must be made for the proper disposal and burying of all remaining tissues from the donor. The Torah (*Deuteronomy* 21:22-23) mandates rapid burial of a dead body: "And if there be a man in sin deserving death, and he be put to death, and you hang him on a tree; his body shall not remain all night upon the tree, but you shall surely bury him that day; for he that is hanged is a reproach to God." This was later codified by R. Caro (Sh Ar, *Yoreh Deah* 357:1). The transplanted organs remain in and are buried with the recipient after death, even if they were implanted into a non-Jew. R. Feinstein (IM, *Yoreh Deah* I, #231) requires the burial of all organs and tissues, while the CJLS (112589) requires burial of amputated limbs, not internal organs or isolated other tissues, in accordance with the opinion of Maimonides (MT, *Hilchot Tumat Hamet* 2:3). A related issue relates to guaranteeing that the donated organs will be used, not wasted. The presumption in these cases is that there exists a *choleh le'faneinu* (sick person immediately before us) who will benefit from the organ, particularly given the current successes with transplantation and the long waiting lists for organs (See **Autopsy** for a more in-depth explanation of the concept of *choleh le'faneinu*). Finally, some have suggested that it is inappropriate for Jews to donate organs because the body will not be intact at the time of the resurrection of the dead (Maimonides' 13th Principle of Faith). This concern is totally invalid because of the belief that a God that is sufficiently powerful to resurrect the dead is capable of resupplying any missing organs.

Mutilation of and deriving benefit from the corpse are closely related in the case of organ donation. Although a principle of "*met assur b'hana'ah*" (benefiting from the dead) (BT, *Sanhedrin* 47b) exists, there is another conflicting Talmudic principle that states, "One may use any materials for healing except those that are associated with idolatry, immorality and murder" (BT, *Pesachim* 25a). Maimonides codified this (MT, *Yesodei HaTorah* 5:6) as "He that is sick and in danger of death, and the doctor tells him that he can be cured by a certain object or material which is forbidden by the Torah, he must obey the doctor and be cured." R. Caro agrees (Sh Ar, *Yoreh Deah* 155:3). Resolution of this conflict hinges upon the definition of *hana'ah* (deriving "benefit" from the dead). Most authorities have understood the notion of *hana'ah* as being similar to the satisfaction associated with eating. Since the use of cadaver organs for transplantation is not analogous to eating, it would be considered "*lo k'derech hanato*" (not in the way of benefit) and therefore permitted (IM, *Yoreh Deah* #229, 230; CJLS 122788, 090777; ARR # 84; CCAR #86).

Some Orthodox authorities, including R. Tendler and the Rabbinical Council of America, have suggested that organ donation should be mandatory because of the commandments "You shall not stand idly by the blood of thy fellow" (*Leviticus* 19:16), "And you shall restore it to him" (*Deuteronomy* 22:2), "Love your neighbor as yourself " (*Leviticus* 19:18), and the Talmudic dictum "All of Israel is responsible one for the other" (BT, *Shevuot* 39a, *Sanhedrin* 73a). Other Orthodox scholars have maintained that organ donation is optional; still others are of the opinion that it is forbidden according to *halacha.* The Committee on Jewish Law and Standards of the Rabbinical Assembly (Conservative Judaism) in 1996 opined that it was mandatory based upon *halacha* for Jews to donate cadaver organs, modifying its earlier positions (113073, 110977) that were strongly supportive. The Bioethics Committee of the Central Conference of American Rabbis (Reform Judaism), concurs in this view that Jews should donate cadaver organs. The CJLS and CCAR also sanction the "banking" of cadaver organs for the purposes of future transplantation (090777, 122788; ARR #84; CARR #78). The CCAR also permits a dying fetus to be kept alive for a brief period for the purpose of donating organs, with appropriate parental permission (NARR #163).

The debate over the question of cadaver organ donation on one level pits the concern for the integrity of the dying person against modern medicine, and, on another, the concern of the integrity of the body of the deceased against the life of the recipient. Both situations illustrate Judaism's commitment to the dignity of mankind when people are most vulnerable.

*Natan's family agrees to the organ donation. The kidney and pancreas are successfully transplanted into Devorah, and the heart, lungs, liver and corneas are sent elsewhere for transplantation. She does well following the transplant and is discharged home after two weeks.*

***Six months later.*** *Devorah's life dramatically improves. Again, she is committed to following carefully all of her doctor's* *orders. She takes her medications with great care. After recovering from surgery, she begins a new job. She would like to begin dating, but is very self-conscious about her appearance. Her self-esteem was badly damaged through her adolescent years and she has little confidence or experience in social situations. She wants to have a rhinoplasty ("nose job"), which she believes will improve the way she looks, and consequently, her self-esteem and social life. Devorah's parents are skeptical about any additional surgery, even elective surgery. They feel as though she has already "been through enough."*

Cosmetic surgery is commonly performed today for a variety of reasons. Although medical treatment is clearly sanctioned in Judaism for situations in which there is a danger to life, it does not subscribe to the notion that individuals have free reign to do as they please with their bodies.

**Issues**: Cosmetic and elective surgery

## Cosmetic and Elective Surgery

Much of cosmetic surgery is generally classified as elective, with no compelling medical reason or physical malady requiring such surgery. Since all surgery, whether optional or minor, involves some risk, the decision to proceed with any diagnostic or therapeutic procedure requires that the potential benefits outweigh the risks. Judaism takes a similar view of elective surgery, which is based upon a variety of sources. First, according to *halacha*, one does not exercise complete dominion over his or her body and therefore must act in accordance with certain principles. As we have already seen, there is a clear prohibition in Judaism against placing oneself in danger based upon several Biblical and Talmudic sources. There is also an injunction against harming or wounding oneself, based upon a statement by R. Akiva (Mishnah, *Bava Kamma* 8:5), which is later codified by Maimonides (MT, *Hilchot Chovel* 5:1), and R. Caro (Sh Ar, *Choshen Mishpat* 420.31). However, *poskim* have been lenient in the area of elective surgery when the risks are minimal (IM, *Choshen Mishpat* #103; NA, *Yoreh Deah* 349,3:3:2, 3:3:3; *Choshen Mishpat* 420:1). Thus, justification for any procedure, elective or otherwise, similarly requires demonstration that the benefits offset the risks.

The question of cosmetic surgery is particularly interesting because considerable attention has been paid to the role of cosmetics and appearance in the Tanach, Talmud and codes of law. The commentators on the *Book of Exodus* (38:8) discuss the importance of appearance of the Jewish women in Egypt in maintaining the morale of the men. The *Megillat Esther* 2:12 and *Song of Songs* 3:6 provide extensive lists of spices that were used to enhance a woman's appearance. The Mishnah (*Yebamot* 9:10) describes the case of a sage beautifying a homely girl for the purpose of marriage. In terms of law, the Talmud (BT, *Ketubot* 64b) requires a husband to provide for his wife's cosmetic needs and the *Shulchan Aruch (Orach Chayim* 346:5) allows for women to partake of beauty treatments on *chol ha'moed,* the intermediate days of a festival.

Cosmetic surgery has generally been sanctioned by *halacha* when two conditions have been met. First, the risk of the procedure must be sufficiently low so that it can be considered that the "masses have trodden upon it" (BT, *Shabbat* 129b). Once this has been established, there must be a tangible gain resulting from the procedure, such as improvement in an individual's financial situation because it becomes easier to earn a living or a psychological benefit because the procedure would relieve emotional distress. Whether a particular rabbi will approve or disapprove of a procedure in any given case will usually depend upon the individual circumstances and his own biases. To some rabbis, the prospect of dating and finding a spouse would represent sufficient psychological stress to justify a rhinoplasty (IM, *Choshen Mishpat* II #66; ARR #172), whereas to others it might not (TE, V, 11#41). The Reform rabbinate addressed the issue of elective breast enlargement involving silicone gel implants. Because of the potential dangers associated with these implants, restraint was advised against cosmetic surgery in the absence of compelling psychological and emotional factors (CARR 5752.7).

The issue of elective surgery highlights the contrast between Judaism's understanding of God's ownership of one's body, and the individual's stewardship and responsibility for the body.

***Two months later.*** *Devorah undergoes a rhinoplasty. She feels better about herself and begins dating. After a few months, she meets and falls in love with a nice young man, Gabriel. Gabriel is willing to marry Devorah despite all of her medical problems. However, his parents are concerned about her illness and long-term prognosis. They would like to discuss* *her medical problems with Devorah's physicians. Devorah is resentful about this intrusion into her private affairs. She feels strongly that these issues are personal, or only between Gabriel and herself.*

The right to privacy is fundamental in Western democracies. This entitlement has been extended to include the sanctity of the relationships between marital partners, doctors and patients, lawyers and clients and clergymen and congregants. Similarly, the strength of each of these relationships is dependent upon the existence of honesty, trust and respect between the parties. How does Jewish tradition view these critical issues?

**Issues**: Confidentiality and truth telling

## Confidentiality and Truth Telling

The Torah contains no specific laws concerning confidentiality. Rather, laws of confidentiality are subsumed under the category of *l'shon hara* (evil speech) and *rechilut* (gossip). "You shall not go as a bearer of tales among your people...." (*Leviticus* 19:16). Numerous religious treatises have been published on the subject of gossip; the best known is by R. Israel Meir Kagan, otherwise known as the Chafetz Chaim.

Every person who attends synagogue regularly has heard speeches from the pulpit railing against the evils and destructiveness of *l'shon hara*. In fact, the commentators recognized the harm that can be inflicted through words and equates *l'shon hara* with murder, since the destruction of a person's reputation can devastate his life.

The *halachot* surrounding *l'shon hara* and *rechilut* differ significantly from those concerning libel and slander under civil law. The major distinction is that dissemination of negative or hurtful information, even if true or said without malice, still constitutes *l'shon hara* (MT, *Hilchot Deot* 7:2). However, there are limits on this seemingly straightforward ban against harmful speech, which can be derived from the second portion of the verse in *Leviticus* 19:16: "... nor shall you stand idly by the blood of your fellow" (referred to as *lo ta'amod*). This statement suggests that the exhortation against telling tales ends at the point where detriment may come to another. Just as it is prohibited to gossip about another individual because it may result in harm, it is equally wrong to withhold certain information if doing so will damage another person. Furthermore, there is a positive commandment (*Leviticus* 5:1) to come forward with information that is beneficial to others, which is also codified in the Talmud (BT, *Bava Kamma* 56a) and Shulchan Aruch (*Choshen Mishpat* 28:1). Thus, the critical issue is whether the disclosure of information will help circumvent physical or emotional injury, loss or damage to property.

The situation may be similar to the case of a *rodef* (pursuer), who must be stopped when posing a threat to the individual. However, if no threat exists or the information in question can be obtained in another manner, then it would be forbidden to reveal any privileged communication. For example, when a police officer is pursuing an armed robber, the use of deadly force is only condoned if the officer's life is directly threatened.

Based upon these considerations, the Chafetz Chaim ruled that under certain circumstances it is permissible to disclose seemingly confidential information, for example, to a potential marriage partner or to someone in danger of being physically harmed. The parameters governing such disclosure are severely restricted. First, there must be the presence of a significant disease or physical defect. Second, the nature or extent of the problem must not be exaggerated when the information is released. Third, the purpose of reporting the facts must only be to benefit the recipient. Last, it must be reasonable to assume the information is critical and will materially affect the outcome. Thus, the *halacha* attempts to balance the interests of the patient against those of others; neither is considered absolute or inviolable.

Recently, ethical questions have been raised about the confidentiality of medical records and the release of personal information to insurance carriers and employers. In the past, such disclosure often centered on psychiatric illnesses, sexually transmitted diseases or abortions. Now, advances in biotechnology have led to the identification of numerous markers indicating a genetic predisposition to such diseases as breast cancer (especially in Ashkenazi women), colon cancer, cystic fibrosis, schizophrenia and depression. Access by employers or insurance companies to such information carries enormous implications. For the individual, job security, insurability and future access to health care may be threatened. For employers and insurers, the availability of such data allows them to make more accurate actuarial estimates and adjust policies accordingly. A balance must be struck between the individual's right to privacy and the other parties' right to truthful and accurate disclosure. The dilemma is accentuated by the fact that a genetic predisposition does not mean that an individual will develop a health problem. Yet, that information may be used to arrive at a decision that adversely affects the person. Guidelines and legislation are currently being developed by professional societies and lawmakers to deal with these questions.

There are halachic concerns regarding this issue. Judaism does not recognize an inherent or absolute right to privacy, as noted above. Based on the principles elucidated by the Chafetz Chaim, it may sometimes be appropriate to disclose personal information if such knowledge will have a material effect on the issue at hand. Also, because Judaism does not recognize such a right, a tension exists between the rights of the individual and the rights of the community. In general, when a conflict arises between the individual and the *kehilla* (community), the *halacha* usually gives priority to the community. For example, R. Waldenberg has ruled that physicians are obligated to testify in court, if necessary, and notify the appropriate authorities in cases where they discover that patients who are driving suffer from conditions such as blindness or epilepsy that endanger public safety (TE, XIII, #81:2, #104:1, XV 13 #1, XVI #4). R. Auerbach has similarly ruled that physicians are bound to report cases of child abuse (NA, *Choshen Mishpat* 388.1). Similarly, divulging confidential information may involve the violation of an oath (Hippocratic or other) taken by a physician. However, R. Waldenberg has argued in such a matter that this is not so, since an observant physician would never have intended to violate Jewish law when taking a professional oath (TE, V 13 #81). A more controversial application of halachic principles would mandate HIV testing and disclosure in all cases where it was advocated by public health experts, regardless of the political ramifications. *Halacha* would require informing a prospective spouse of his or her intended partner's HIV status (NA, *Even HaEzer* 2:1:1; 2:1:2), a policy that differs considerably from current American law. However, it is not at all clear whether *halacha* would apply in a case of disclosure to a corporate entity, such as an employer, insurance company or government agency. The Reform rabbinate has issued several responsa dealing with questions of confidentiality that are generally consistent with traditional views (CARR #5; CCARR 5750.3, 5753.2; 5756.2).

Closely related to confidentiality is the issue of truth telling. Truth telling differs from confidentiality in that it involves the caregiver's obligation to disclose information to the patient, or others, honestly and in a timely manner. In other words, truth telling deals with what information is provided, whereas confidentiality refers to the recipient of the information.

The Torah contains numerous admonitions against lying that encompass a wide variety of circumstances. "Thou shall not utter a false report" (*Exodus* 23:1) and "Thou shall not bear false witness" (*Exodus* 20:13) deal with the prohibition against perjury, while "Thou shall not render a false judgment" (*Exodus* 23:6) and "Distance yourself from a matter of falsehood" (*Exodus* 23:7) apply to judges. Concerning business dealings, the Torah states: "Neither shall you deal falsely, nor lie to one another" (*Leviticus* 19:11) and "You shall not commit a perversion in justice, in measures of length, weight or volume" (*Leviticus* 19:35). Even the appearance of impropriety in any of these areas is strongly condemned. Other scriptural exhortations against lying appear in *Proverbs:* ("Lying lips are an abomination to the Lord" [12:22]) and *Psalms*, where King David states, "He that speaks falsely shall not appear before my eyes" (101:7). The Talmud also contains several negative comments about lying: "The liar is like an idolater" (BT, *Sanhedrin* 92a) and "Falsehood is frequent, truth is rare" (BT, *Shabbat* 104a). Even self-serving, although harmless deception, known as *g'neivat da'at* (literally: theft of knowledge) is also prohibited.

Despite these unequivocal condemnations of lying, the Talmud rules: "You may modify a statement in the interests of peace" (BT, *Yebamot* 65b, also *Ketubot* 17a, *Bava Metzia* 23b). Thus, the *halacha* permits telling a "white lie" on occasion in order to maintain *shalom bayit* (peaceful marital relations) and avoid physical or emotional pain, anguish, and embarrassment. In this regard, the Sages took a clear position against increasing the psychological or emotional stress of seriously or terminally ill patients because of the fear of *tiruf hada'at* (emotional shock) that could potentially aggravate their condition or shorten their lives. The Talmud (BT, *Moed Katan* 26b) forbids informing a seriously ill person about the death of a close relative or friend. This was later codified by R. Caro (Sh Ar, *Yoreh Deah* 337). More recently, R. Feinstein (IM, *Choshen Mishpat* II, #73:2) reiterated the importance of not increasing the mental anguish of a dying patient by inappropriate or insensitive words or actions.

Obviously a balance must be struck between the need to provide patients with honest and necessary appraisal of the situation and the avoidance of serious emotional and psychological harm that may aggravate their physical condition. Certainly, physicians are required to be open and veracious with their patients in the early stages of any illness, so that proper informed decisions about available treatment options can be made. Similarly, patients need, and are entitled, to set their affairs in order and make necessary plans for the well being and care of their families and assets. There is no conflict between Jewish tradition and contemporary ethicists that advocate complete disclosure under any circumstances as a fundamental right and obligation. While Jewish tradition endorses honesty as a virtue and deplores deception, it also recognizes the potential for harm to individuals in a fragile state of mind, especially those with terminal conditions. Here, physicians are cautioned to avoid giving unnecessary information that may precipitate depression or hasten death and are encouraged to provide comfort and solace, maintaining a sense of hope in the face of despair. In the High Holy Day liturgy we say: "*U'teshuvah, u'tefillah, u'tzedakah, ma'averin et roah ha'gezeirah*" ("Repentance, prayer and charity may overturn the negative decree"). The importance of physicians exercising discretion is reinforced in several Reform responsa (ARR #74; CARR 5753.2; 5756.2) and by Rabbis Tendler and Bleich and Drs. A.S. Abraham and F. Rosner.

Judaism's understanding of truth telling and confidentiality is based upon the importance that our choice of words plays within society. It further exemplifies the priority that *halacha* gives to the welfare of the community over the rights of its individual members.

## Chapter 6: ISSUES OF PROCREATION AND ABORTION

*One year later. Devorah and Gabriel marry. After a year, they contemplate starting a family. They discuss this with Devorah's doctors, who voice concern about the stress of pregnancy on Devorah and the chances of her children developing diabetes or some other genetic problems because of the immunosuppressive medications she is taking. The situation is further complicated because there is a questionable history of Tay-Sachs disease (a uniformly fatal, genetically transmitted disease that affects Ashkenazi Jews) in Gabriel's family. The doctors are highly skeptical and advise them to postpone children for awhile because of their fear that pregnancy could exacerbate Devorah's medical condition and compromise the viability of her transplant. The couple is advised to utilize birth control in the meantime; the doctors have even suggested that they contemplate sterilization.*

*Devorah does not want to see any child of hers suffer as she has. However, all of her friends are having babies and she feels that she does not want to miss experiencing pregnancy and motherhood. She is constantly sad and cannot get the idea of having a baby out of her mind.*

Sexuality is an integral component of the marital relationship, not only as part of a couple's desire for children, but because of its contribution toward the emotional and psychological health of the couple.

**Issues**: Jewish Attitude Toward Sex and Sexuality
The Obligation for Procreation
Genetic Counseling and Screening
Contraception

**Jewish Attitude Toward Sex and Sexuality**

In Jewish tradition, sex is best discussed within the context of marriage, a union which is viewed as the ideal and in which sex is recognized as a normal component. The Hebrew word for marriage is *kiddushin*, whose root is the word *kadosh*, meaning holy. For these reasons, marriage, sexuality and procreation are strongly promoted in Judaism.

Judaism considers marriage so central to the human condition that the Torah introduces it in the creation story (*Genesis* 2:18, 24): "It is not good for man to be alone; I will make for him a helpmate....Therefore, shall a man leave his father and his mother, and cleave to his wife, and they shall be one flesh." The Rabbis and commentators repeatedly emphasized the companionship aspect of marriage, condemning celibacy. "A man without a wife is considered incomplete" (Midrash, *Genesis Rabbah* 17:2). "He who remains unmarried is without joy, blessing, good, Torah, protection and peace" (BT, *Yebamot* 62b). "A man who remains unmarried is without life" (BT, *Yebamot* 64b). Concerning women's needs, the Talmud advances a positive opinion of marriage (BT, *Yebamot* 118b): "It is always to her advantage to be married rather than be alone." One of the most lovely passages reflecting the Jewish view of the beauty and holiness of marriage is found in the *Midrash* (*Genesis Rabbah* 8:9): "No man without woman; no woman without man; and neither together without the Almighty."

Equally prominent in Biblical and Talmudic literature are condemnations of illicit sexual relationships outside of marriage, emphasizing the importance of morality over sexuality. These include censure of casual sex as well as forbidden relationships. "If a man finds a virgin who was not betrothed and lies with her, and they are found, then the man shall pay to the father of the maiden fifty silver pieces, and she shall be his wife because he afflicted her; he can never divorce her all his life" (*Deuteronomy* 22:28-29). The prohibition against adultery (*Exodus* 20:13) is well known and the punishments for it described in detail (*Numbers* 5:12-31); furthermore, an entire tractate of the Babylonian Talmud, *Sotah*, is devoted to this subject. These concerns led to numerous restrictions on the behavior of men and women in Talmudic and post-Talmudic times. Men were forbidden to walk behind women, hear their voices or look at their hair (BT, *B'rachot* 24a, 61a). Even the thought of an illicit relationship was condemned: "Do not consider only a man who sins with his body an adulterer, it applies even to one who also sins with his eyes" (*Vayikra Rabbah* 23). Numerous other restrictions were enacted to ensure the physical separation of men and women, both single and married, in a host of situations, including prayer, in business dealings and on social occasions (BT, *Sukkah* 51b; MT, *Hilchot Yom Tov* 6:21; Sh Ar, *Even HaEzer* 21). These prohibitions have been met with much resistance within modern Western civilization. Despite a greater relaxation of standards in this area, the Conservative and Reform movements have each formally confirmed the sanctity of marriage in Judaism and frowned upon casual sexual relations (Dorff E.N., "This is my Beloved, This is My Friend": A Rabbinic Letter on Intimate Relations, 1996; ARR #154).

Not only is sex necessary for procreation, it is conducive to maintaining *shalom bayit* (marital peace) and enhancing the emotional bond between partners. Humans are unique among the species in that they have the ability to engage in sex based upon emotions and intellect rather than by instinct, have sex at times other than during their fertile periods and can face each other during sexual intercourse. Sexuality is recognized in Jewish tradition as a natural drive that must be properly tempered and controlled in order not to be abused. Maimonides emphasized this point (MT, *Hilchot Deot* 4) when he discussed the interrelationship between sexuality and physical health. The Talmud (BT, *Kiddushin* 30b) regards sex as a holy act and considers God a partner to the father and the mother in human creation. Much of the kabbalistic *Zohar* (major work of Jewish mysticism) and the *Song of Songs* utilize sexually explicit metaphors to describe the relationship between God and Israel.

Further evidence supports the intrinsic value placed upon sexuality within marriage, as distinguished from sex for the purpose of procreation. Judaism does not forbid marriage and sexual relations between sterile partners or sexual activity that cannot result in pregnancy (Rama on Sh Ar, *Even HaEzer* 1:3; IM, *Even HaEzer* 63, 67). In the event that a woman is incapable of conceiving, her husband is still obliged to have sexual relations with her to satisfy the commandment of *onah* (Rama on Sh Ar, *Even HaEzer* 154:10). Although there are Biblical (*Deuteronomy* 23:2) and Talmudic (BT, *Yebamot* 75b, 76a) prohibitions against marriage to men with injured genital organs, Rabbis Waldenberg and Feinstein have ruled that such unions are permissible.

The Jewish tradition's positive approach to sexuality is formalized by the elevation of the sex act between marriage partners to the category of *mitzvah* (positive religious obligation). The specific *mitzvot* pertaining to sex involve procreation (see below), *onah* (the halachic obligation for a husband to sexually satisfy his wife) and the laws of *tohorat hamishpacha* (family purity). The requirement of a husband to provide his wife with sexual pleasure (*onah*) is unique to Judaism, which may be one of the few cultures in the world that gives priority to the women's sexual needs over the man's. Thus, women are encouraged to initiate sexual contact and are granted conjugal rights while men are obligated to fulfill their conjugal responsibilities and are forbidden to force themselves on their wives (MT, *Hilchot Ishut* 14:2,7;15:1,16,17,19; Sh Ar, *Even HaEzer* 25:2). A husband's obligation to "honor, feed and support" a wife and "provide food, clothing, necessities of life and conjugal needs" (*Exodus* 21:10) is stipulated in the *ketubah* (marriage contract). Considerable leeway is granted to the couple in terms of how they choose to engage in sex (BT, *Yebamot* 20b; MT, *Hilchot Issurei Biah* 21:9; Sh Ar, *Even HaEzer* 25:2).

The sexual relationship between partners is limited by the laws of *tohorat hamishpacha* (family purity) and the prohibition against *hashchatat zera l'vatalah* (improper discharge of sperm or "onanism"). The laws of *tohorat hamishpacha*, which forbid physical contact between husband and wife during, and for a week following her menstrual period until she immerses herself in a *mikvah* (ritual bath), can be understood from a practical perspective. This cycle encourages sexual relations at the time of ovulation, which maximizes the chance of conception. Forbidding a couple to have sexual relations for about two weeks each month also facilitates the nurturing and development of a strong emotional and intellectual bond between husband and wife. Such a relationship is alluded to in the *sheva b'rachot* (seven blessings) that accompany the wedding ceremony, where the couple is described as *rayim ahuvim* (loving companions).

Judaism has historically displayed a negative attitude toward forbidden sexual relationships, such as homosexuality, incest, bestiality and acts such as masturbation. The Torah clearly states (*Leviticus* 18:22, 23): "You shall not lie together with a man as with a woman, it is an abomination. Do not lie with an animal to be contaminated with it; nor shall a woman stand before an animal for mating, it is an abomination." The disapproval of homosexuality is well-rooted in Jewish law (MT, *Hilchot Issurei Biah* 1:14; *Hilchot Melachim* 9:5-6). Homosexuality is regarded as a grave sin, perverting one of the fundamental purposes of mankind, procreation (known as *p'ru ur'vu*) and populating the world (known as *la'shevet*) and undermining the moral fabric of marriage and society. Nevertheless, the negative viewpoint toward homosexuality must be distinguished from the treatment accorded to gays and lesbians. All individuals are created in the image of God and deserve to be treated with dignity and respect. We are taught: "There is no death without sin, no suffering without transgression" (BT, *Shabbat* 55a) and that "there is no righteous person on earth who does good and will not sin" (*Ecclesiastes* 7:20). Therefore, it is inappropriate for people to judge others or to make them feel unwelcome within the community (ARR #13,14). Nevertheless, this traditional prohibition against homosexuality, according to all Orthodox authorities and a number of more traditional Conservative (Kimmelman) and Reform thinkers (CCAR #201), remains immutable even in the face of new evidence suggesting that homosexuality may be predetermined genetically and, therefore, is not a choice of lifestyle. This view maintains that even if homosexuality is the result of, or heavily influenced by, "nature," these mitigating factors serve only to lessen or even eliminate any culpability, but do not obviate the underlying religious prohibition.

More liberal Conservative (R. Dorff) and Reform thinkers have advocated a re-evaluation of the traditional position, arguing that our understanding of homosexuality and the nature of family relationships within society have changed. In the past, homosexuality was practiced promiscuously in cults and other licentious settings; it was those acts that were traditionally condemned. This is no longer the case, with many homosexuals living in loving, monogamous relationships and forming family units. Homosexuals may now parent children obtained through adoption or advanced reproductive technologies. Also, because homosexuality may have a strong biological and genetic component, homosexuals cannot justifiably be condemned for their behavior. Finally, it is "un-Jewish" to believe that God would proscribe a behavior over which people had no control. Thus, attitudes toward homosexuality within various segments of the Jewish community continue to evolve.

Masturbation has historically been viewed negatively by Jewish tradition, which prohibits the discharge of sperm "in vain" (*hashchatat zera l'vatalah).* This prohibition, known as "onanism," is based upon the Biblical story of Er and Onan (*Genesis* 38:9-19), in which Judah's son, Onan, refused to carry out his obligation of levirate marriage to Tamar and ejaculated on the ground, for which he was subsequently punished by death. Maimonides (MT, *Hilchot Issurei Bi'ah* 21:18) expressly forbids masturbation: "It is forbidden to emit semen for no purpose. Thus, a man should not move within and ejaculate outside.... As to those who masturbate, they commit a forbidden act....it is regarded as they have killed a human being." R. Caro concurs (Sh Ar, *Even HaEzer* 21:5). In Mishneh Torah (*Hilchot Deot* 4:19), Maimonides expounds upon his understanding of the negative effects of male sexual excess: "Semen is the strength of the body, its light and the light of its eyes. Excessive emission leads to physical decay, debility and decreased vitality.... Whoever engages in excessive sexual emission ages prematurely, his strength fails, his eyes become dim...Medical authorities have stated that for each person who dies of other maladies, a thousand are victims of sexual excess." In addition, there are issues of ritual impurity related to male emissions just as there are to female menstruation.

While Judaism clearly endorses the idea that sexual relations should be confined to marriage, R. Dorff, a Conservative authority, notes that many young people will be sexually active outside of marriage. Given the risks posed by sexually transmitted disease, masturbation may be preferable to, or less objectionable than, non-marital intercourse, even with the use of contraception. R. Dorff also points out that traditionally, the objection to masturbation is applied to men, not women, since there is no emission of "seed" involved for the latter.

Human companionship and procreation are recognized by Jewish tradition through its elevation of marriage and sex to acts of holiness. The specific role played by each is emphasized in order to achieve true personal fulfillment as well as to guarantee the perpetuation of the Jewish people.

**The Obligation for Procreation**

The requirement to procreate is based upon three sources, one Biblical and two Rabbinic. After the great flood, the Torah (*Genesis* 9:7) records that God commanded Noah and his sons: "...be fruitful and multiply [*p'ru ur'vu*] and bring forth abundantly in the earth, and multiply in it." The Talmud (BT, *Yebamot* 63b) expounds on this: "He who does not engage in procreation is as if he has committed murder." The requirement to reproduce is further clarified in the Mishnah (*Yebamot* 6:6): "A man shall not abstain from performing the duty of propagating the race unless he already has two children. Beit Shammai ruled two males and Beit Hillel ruled a male and a female, based upon the verse 'male and female He created them' (*Genesis* 1:27). The law is according to Hillel." This is codified in the *Shulchan Aruch* (*Even HaEzer* 1:5).

The Rabbinic sources in this area, known as *la'shevet* (to inhabit) and *la'erev* (in the twilight), are derived from two other verses in the Tanach. In response to the statement by the prophet Isaiah (45:18), "For thus says the Lord, Creator of the Heavens: He is the God who formed the earth and made it, He did not create it for void - He formed it to be inhabited (*la'shevet*)," the Talmud (BT, *Chagigah* 2b) states, "Was not the world created for propagation?" Furthermore, King Solomon wrote (*Ecclesiastes* 11:6), "In the morning sow your seed, and in the evening do not withhold your hand, because you do not know from which will prosper..." This was interpreted (BT, *Yebamot* 65b) to mean "if a man had children in his youth, he should also have children in his old age (*la'erev*)." Maimonides later codified this (MT, *Hilchot Ishut* 15:16) as: "Although a man has fulfilled the commandment to procreate, he is still commanded by the Rabbis not to refrain from procreating as long as he still has strength. Anyone who adds a soul to the Jewish people is considered as though he added an entire world."

Other evidence supporting the commandment to reproduce includes permission to sell a Torah scroll, which is forbidden under other circumstances, in order to acquire money to marry and have children (BT, *Megillah* 27a). Similarly, a *Kohen* living in the land of Israel, normally prohibited from leaving the country, is allowed to move elsewhere for the purpose of marriage and starting a family (BT, *Avodah Zarah* 13a). Provisions also exist in the Talmud (BT, *Ta'anit* 31a, *Yebamot* 2b) for dissolving a marriage in the event that one of the partners is unwilling or incapable of having children, although divorce under these circumstances is not required. Thus, it is clear that there is strong Biblical and Rabbinic opinion in support of a duty to reproduce.

Despite this clear emphasis on procreation, the Rabbis have interpreted this Biblical obligation to be incumbent only on men, not women. The Talmud (BT, *Yebamot* 65b) states that the commandment to "increase and multiply, and fill the earth..." applies only to one whose nature is to subdue it -- that is, to man, who by nature is more aggressive. Women are more naturally considered to be bound by the *mitzvah* of *la'shevet,* populating the world. Despite this inclination, the commentator Meshech Chochmah (*Genesis* 9:1), says that women are not required to have children because childbirth endangers their lives, and one cannot be forced to place oneself in a perilous situation. By having children, though, women perform a *mitzvah* because they enable their husbands to fulfill the commandment. "The act of the enabler is even greater than the one who does it" (BT, *Bava Batra* 9a). [Halachic permission for women to assume the risk of pregnancy and childbirth is based upon the concept of "the masses have trodden upon it" (BT, *Shabbat* 129b)].

Although the need for reproduction has universal implications for the human race, the specific commandment applies to Jews. For example, converts to Judaism are considered to have fulfilled this *mitzvah* if their children convert to Judaism as well (MT, *Hilchot Ishut* 15:6). Some authorities believe adopting and raising a child as a Jew partially fulfills this obligation.

A related issue concerns family planning. A Talmudic principle, *z'rizim makdimim l'mitzvot* (zealously performing *mitzvot* at the earliest possible time) (BT, *Pesachim* 4a), is also applicable to the commandment of procreation. This is codified by Maimonides (MT, *Hilchot Ishut* 15:1) and R. Caro (Sh Ar *Even HaEzer* 76:6). Only in extenuating circumstances, such as where the husband is involved in Torah study, is the postponement of procreation sanctioned based on the principle that one engaged in the performance of a *mitzvah* is exempt from other *mitzvot* (MT, *Hilchot Ishut* 15:2). In modern times, exemptions by Orthodox authorities have been granted in situations where pregnancy or childbirth would pose a significant physical or emotional risk to the mother (IM, *Even HaEzer* I #63, IV #62, #67, 69; NA *Even HaEzer* 5:13), or to ensure *shalom bayit* (domestic tranquility) (IM, *Even HaEzer* II #71, IV #73). Similar positions have been advanced by Conservative scholar R. Ben Zion Bokser (1961) and R. Jacob of the Reform movement (ARR #156), emphasizing the importance of the wife's perception of her own emotional health based upon the adage: "The heart knows its own bitterness" (*Proverbs* 14:10).

The commandment to procreate is part of Jewish law. By considering this to be a religious obligation and a holy act performed in partnership with God, the Sages took a powerful step toward ensuring the future of the Jewish people.

**Genetic Counseling and Screening**

Advances in the study of human genetics have increased the worth and utility of genetic screening and counseling. Current techniques in molecular biology make it possible to evaluate individuals for potential hereditary disorders and to examine the genetic composition of embryos and fetuses. In the past, interest in this type of screening and counseling within the Jewish community has centered around identification of potential carriers and prevention of such inherited diseases as Tay-Sachs, Familial Dysautonomia and Gaucher's, which predominantly affect the central nervous system of Ashkenazi Jews, and Thalassemia Major and Minor, two congenital forms of anemia that primarily afflict Sephardic Jews. In addition to their impact on the victims, who frequently die a premature death, these illnesses can be devastating to their families, resulting in severe psychological trauma, grief and guilt on the part of the parents.

The halachic concerns regarding genetic screening and counseling relate to the context in which they are performed, the ultimate goal of the screening process and the impact of the information on the individuals in question. Most halachic authorities find testing permissible if it is done prior to marriage in order to inform a person of his status as a carrier of a particular disease, or to prevent a marriage to another carrier. Appropriate safeguards guaranteeing confidentiality must be maintained, however, and psychological support must also be available (IM, *Even HaEzer* IV #10).

After marriage, however, most rabbinic authorities do not sanction screening if the results will lead to childless unions. Most Orthodox rabbinic authorities (IM, *Choshen Mishpat* II #71; NA, *Choshen Mishpat* 425:1:15), with the exception of R. Waldenberg (TE IX #236, 327, XIII #102), disapprove of genetic screening after marriage if identification of one's carrier status would lead to monitoring a pregnancy through amniocentesis -- and, if the fetus is affected -- abortion. Conservative and Reform rabbis are generally more lenient in this regard, allowing amniocentesis and possibly abortion, especially if it is determined that the child will be born severely defective or if the birth of such a child will have a significantly negative effect on the psychological well-being of the parents, particularly the mother

(Proceedings of the CJLS 1980-1985; ARR #171; CARR #16; RRR #41; NARR #155). The yardstick employed by different rabbis is extremely variable and each case must be considered individually and decided upon its own merits. To some, the possibility of being pregnant with a severely retarded fetus may justify amniocentesis, whereas to others, it may not.

Newer biochemical techniques of DNA analysis can determine the sex of offspring and screen for genetic abnormalities at a much earlier developmental stage. For couples undergoing in vitro fertilization as treatment for infertility, this technique can be accomplished even before implantation, thus avoiding the use of any genetically defective embryos or embryos that may harbor an identifiable congenital defect or a sex-linked genetic disease (such as hemophilia). In this situation, many authorities would allow genetic screening because the unimplanted embryos have no status according to *halacha*, and therefore may be destroyed (NA, *Even HaEzer* 1:1). More complicated are issues related to the identification of genes that signal a predisposition to certain conditions such as breast or colon cancer -- which may or may not affect the offspring later in life. Generally, such possibilities, or even probabilities, are not considered valid halachic reasons for aborting a fetus unless they have a severe psychological impact on the mother. In each case, the decision must be individualized by the rabbi, carefully weighing all of the factors involved.

The issue of genetic screening challenges the uniqueness and value of all human life, regardless of form or intelligence. Its resolution according to *halacha* requires that this level of sanctity and respect be maintained.

**Contraception**

Judaism recognizes sexuality as a natural aspect of human existence. This is exemplified by the elevation of the sexual act to the status of a *mitzvah* (*onah*), irrespective of its role in the *mitzvah* of *p'ru u'r'vu* (be fruitful and multiply).

The halachic discussion of contraception involves two distinct issues: the legality of the use of contraception and the permissibility of a particular contraceptive method. The Talmud *(BT, Yebamot 65b)* recognizes the legitimacy of contraception, even sterilization, for a woman because the *mitzvah* of procreation is only incumbent upon a man. The wife of the Sage R. Chiyya experienced considerable difficulty and pain during childbirth and surreptitiously asked her husband if women were obligated to perform this commandment. After being told that they were not, she immediately drank a potion that caused her to become sterile. This practice has subsequently been codified by Maimonides (MT, *Hilchot Issurei Biah* 16:12), R. Caro (Sh Ar, *Even HaEzer* 5:12) and others as a way of establishing the halachic permissibility of birth control. However, despite its legality, birth control has generally been frowned upon in the absence of extenuating circumstances because of the value ascribed to procreation.

In another instance, the Talmud (BT, *Yebamot* 12b) specifically discusses the use of a contraceptive device in what is known commonly as the *Baraita of the Three Women*, upon which virtually all subsequent decisions about contraception are based. [A *baraita* is a an opinion quoted in the Gemara from the Mishnaic period that was not included by R. Judah the Prince in the formal redaction of the Mishnah. Its halachic authority is equivalent to that of the Mishnah.]

> "Three women may [must] use a contraceptive tampon (Hebrew: *moch*) in their marital intercourse: a minor, a pregnant woman, and a nursing mother. The minor

> because she might become pregnant and die. A pregnant woman because she might cause her fetus to become a sandal (fishlike fetus which will be aborted). A nursing woman because she might wean her child prematurely causing its death...This is the opinion of R. Meir. But the Sages say that the one and the other have marital intercourse in the usual way, and mercy will come from Heaven [to save them] as the Bible says, "The Lord preserves the simple (*Psalms* 116:6)."

In this instance, the Talmud decided the law in accordance with the opinion of the Sages, who represent the majority. However, the precise meaning of this passage is disputed with regard to both the permissibility of contraception and the methodology involved in the use of the contraceptive device (*moch*). Concerning the legitimacy of contraception, Rashi interprets the *baraita* as do the Sages, meaning that each of the three types of women mentioned by R. Meir *may* use contraception; which then implies that other women, who are not at increased risk from pregnancy, may not. In contrast, Rabbeinu Tam (a Tosafist and the grandson of Rashi) interprets the *baraita* more broadly, arguing that Meir is saying that those women who fit these circumstances *must* use contraception, while the Sages say that other women merely have the option of doing so. According to Rabbeinu Tam, Rashi's view is incorrect because it is illogical to suggest that the Sages would have forbidden women whose health was at risk to use contraceptives.

The implications of these two interpretations of the *baraita* on the *halacha* are dramatic, and opinions vary depending upon which view a particular decisor subscribes to. Most *Rishonim* and *Achronim* accepted the logic of Rabbeinu Tam's view, based upon the assumption that the Sages would consider the requirement to avoid unnecessary risk paramount. Some of those, such as Asheri and R. Solomon Luria, were lenient and advocated the liberal use of contraceptives by any woman, while other *Rishonim*, including Rashba, Rosh and Ravid, tried to preserve Rashi's reluctance to allow the widespread use of birth control *carte blanche*. In recent years, halachic authorities have issued numerous responsa dealing with the subject of contraception. R. Feinstein published over 25 responsa on this topic.

In general, the decision to allow the use of birth control depends upon the potentially adverse effects of a pregnancy or birth on the couple. Medical reasons in which pregnancy or childbirth would pose a significant physical or emotional risk to the mother are usually considered valid (IM, *Even HaEzer* I #63, IV #62, #67, 69; NA, *Even HaEzer* 5:13, B.Z. Bokser 1961; AAR #156). Some authorities also permit birth control in circumstances where the parents desire to put space between children in order to ensure domestic tranquility (*shalom bayit*), and/or if they are incapable of adequately raising several small children at once (IM, *Even HaEzer* II #71, IV #73; BZ Bokser 1961; AAR #156). Contraception is frowned upon when it is used for social or financial convenience or because of a fear that a child may be born defective, unless these anxieties will result in significant emotional distress. Permission to use contraceptives is usually granted for a prescribed period of time, after which the situation is carefully reassessed to determine whether the precipitating circumstances have changed (IM, *Even HaEzer* I #64). R. Bokser's Conservative responsum (CJLS 1927-70, pp1451-1458) stresses that it is important to carefully consider the mother's own assessment of the effect of the pregnancy on her psychological well-being, based upon the principle "The heart knows its own bitterness" (*Proverbs* 14:10). R. Bokser also points out that in situations in which birth control will be employed, it is halachically preferable for the woman to use it, since the biblical obligation to procreate applies only to the man.

In situations where birth control is utilized, a halachic hierarchy can be formulated based upon the understanding of the *moch*, the degree to which each method interferes with the fulfillment of the *mitzvah* of *onah,* and its effect on the sperm (because of the prohibition against *hashchatat zera l'vatalah* [the improper discharge or destruction of sperm "in vain"]). Here too, the controversy stems from a disagreement between Rashi and Rabbeinu Tam regarding the meaning of the *baraita.* According to Rashi, the *moch* is placed in the woman's body before coitus in order to absorb the sperm and prevent fertilization. Rabbeinu Tam believes that insertion of the *moch* before intercourse renders the act improper (*de'ein derech tashmish*) by violating the requirements of *onah* and the prohibition against *hashchatat zera l'vatalah,* and therefore, must be inserted following intercourse in order to remove the sperm from the vaginal canal. While most *Rishonim* and *Achronim* agreed with Rashi and permitted the use of either precoital or postcoital devices, several influential *Achronim*, R. Akiva Eiger,

R. Moses Sofer (Chatam Sofer) and R. Jacob Ettlinger, strongly opposed the use of any precoital contraceptive devices.

The technical requirements for fulfillment of *onah* are derived from the Biblical verse (*Genesis* 2:24) "Therefore shall a man leave his father and mother and cleave unto his wife, and they shall be one flesh." Thus, the critical issue relates to the term "one flesh," which has been interpreted as mandating physical contact between the parties and the derivative prohibition against the presence of any physical barrier between them. As a result, contraceptive methods that impede total contact between partners, such as a condom, are not acceptable according to all authorities. Regarding a diaphragm, Rabbis C. Sofer (Resp. Machaneh Chaim #53), Feinstein (IM, *Even HaEzer* I #63, II #12, III #21, IV #67-69) and Waldenberg (TE X #25:10) have posited that a diaphragm does not interfere with the commandment of *onah* and is permitted under certain circumstances.

As for the effect of a particular birth control method on the sperm, Judaism forbids the improper discharge or destruction of sperm "in vain" (*hashchatat zera l'vatalah)*. This prohibition of "onanism," derived from the actions of Onan (*Genesis* 38:9-19), is an example of *coitus interruptus*. Maimonides (MT, *Hilchot Issurei Bi'ah* 21:18) specifically forbids this: "It is forbidden to emit semen for no purpose. Thus, a man should not move within and ejaculate outside.... As to those who masturbate, they commit a forbidden act.... it is regarded as they have killed a human being." The Shulchan Aruch (*Even HaEzer* 21:5) concurs.

Regarding *hashchatat zera l'vatalah,* the definition of "in vain" is critical. Most authorities posit that the prohibition against destroying sperm only applies to men, so that birth control methods used by women that involve the destruction or inactivation of sperm may be permissible. Many believe that this prohibition refers only to the physical destruction of the sperm or the use of a mechanical barrier, while others state that physiologic interference, such as with a spermicide, is not allowed. In general, use of birth control methods by men is a greater concern than for women since the commandment for procreation and the prohibition against *hashchatat zera l'vatalah* applies only to men. Despite the problems associated with the use of contraceptives by men, in some cases in which a woman's physical or mental health is threatened, such as from the use of contraceptive pills, the use of condoms has been allowed (IM, *Even HaEzer* I #63, TE XX #50).

Based upon these interpretations, a hierarchy can be established for specific birth control methods currently in use. From the least to most acceptable, the methods are as follows. Condoms are the least acceptable of all methods since they interfere with *onah,* by placing a physical barrier between the partners, and violate the prohibition against *hashchatat zera l'vatalah.* Abstinence is unacceptable because it interferes with the fulfillment of *onah. Coitus interruptus* is forbidden because it violates the prohibition against *hashchatat zera l'vatalah.* A diaphragm may interfere with *onah* by placing a physical barrier between the partners and, if used with a spermicide, may violate the prohibition against *hashchatat zera l'vatalah.* Spermicides may violate the prohibition against *hashchatat zera l'vatalah*, but do not interfere with *onah.* Use of a cervical cap and post-coital removal of semen via a douche or tampon do not interfere with *onah*, but violate the prohibition against *hashchatat zera l'vatalah.* Intrauterine Devices (IUDs) do not interfere with the *onah* (although some rabbis consider the string a barrier) nor do they destroy sperm. They do present halachic problems, nevertheless, because they are believed to function by inducing abortion, have associated medical complications and frequently cause spotting, which affects the status of *niddah* (ritual impurity). Hormonal implants or oral contraceptive pills are the most acceptable contraceptives from a halachic perspective because they neither interfere with *onah* nor destroy sperm (IM, *Even HaEzer* II #17, IV #72,74; NA, *Even HaEzer* 5:13). The problems associated with oral contraceptives primarily relate to their medical complications and issues related to breakthrough bleeding, which affects one's *niddah* status. In recent years, with improvements in the "pill," these risks have been minimized. Sterilization as a method of birth control for men is halachically unacceptable based on a specific Biblical prohibition against castration: "And that which is mauled or crushed or torn or cut you shall not offer to the Lord; nor should you do this in your land" (*Leviticus* 22:24). This prohibition, affirmed by all branches of Judaism (CCAR #198), applies to people as well as animals, and even in circumstances where a man is already known to be infertile (IM, *Even HaEzer* IV #28-31). The only exceptions would be medical necessity (IM, *Even HaEzer* IV #28,29). The CJLS has sanctioned sterilization for men with serious medical conditions who have fulfilled the requirement for procreation (081149, 123149, 040154); however, it is preferable for a woman to use contraceptives rather than for a man to undergo sterilization (051955). For women, sterilization, although less desirable halachically because of its permanence and because women are still obligated in the *mitzvah* of *la'shevet* (IM, *Even HaEzer* III #12,13), may be permissible in rare situations when other forms of contraception are contraindicated (IM, *Even HaEzer* I #13; IV #34, 36). Permission to employ contraceptive methods within Jewish law is based upon a balance between the obligation to perpetuate the human race and the Jewish people and the physical and emotional well-being of parents charged with raising those children.

*Devorah and Gabriel's circumstances appear to have calmed down and stabilized. After a year, they are still interested in having a child. They finally obtain permission from her physicians, although with much reluctance. Unfortunately, it is difficult for Devorah to conceive because of her diabetes and numerous medications. Gabriel is willing to consider adoption, but Devorah is obsessed with the idea of having a biological child. She wants to finally do something "normal" in her life. The couple, particularly Devorah, are anxious to pursue advanced methods of infertility treatment to assist with conception.*

Infertility affects a significant number of couples. New reproductive technologies have enabled many of them to have children, alleviating much of their emotional suffering. At the same time, these advanced methods have raised complex ethical and social issues, with religious implications.

**Issues**: Adoption
Infertility treatment
Advanced reproductive technology
Surrogate motherhood
Cloning

## Adoption

Adoption, *per se*, is not discussed in the Talmud or codes of Jewish law. Yet a strong tradition exists concerning the raising of orphans by people other than their biological parents. The Torah describes Pharaoh's daughter, Batya, rearing Moses (*Exodus* 2:1-10) and admonishes us to care for orphans (*Exodus* 22:20,

*Deuteronomy* 24:17-22). At the end of the *Book of Ruth* (4:7), the special relationship between Naomi, the grandmother, and Ruth's child, Obed, is described: "And her neighbors gave it [the child] a name, saying a son was born to Naomi." When the Talmud (BT, *Sanhedrin* 19b) discusses these two cases, it comments on the fact that Yocheved and Ruth, the birth mothers of Moses and Obed, are not mentioned when referring to their children. The Talmudic discussion concludes: "Whoever raises an orphan in his house is considered as though he has begotten him" and "He who teaches his friend's son Torah is as though he has begotten him." The Midrash (*Sh'mot Rabbah* 4) considers adoption to be an act of *chesed* (loving-kindness) of the highest order and consequently obligates the adoptee to display the greatest level of respect for the parent who raised him. As a result, the material possessions of a minor adopted child go to their adoptive rather than their biological parents (perhaps as partial compensation for the expenses incurred in childrearing). Similarly, in cases where a teacher has raised a child, the codes acknowledge this relationship by giving the teacher priority over a father in certain situations. Lastly, R. Moses Sofer ruled that adopted children are obligated to mourn only for their adopted, not their biological parents.

Despite the above positive portrayal of adoption in the Jewish tradition, it is accompanied with certain halachic conditions. In contrast to adoptions in Western society, in which all legal ties to the biological parents are severed, according to *halacha*, the relationship between an adopted Jewish child and his or her biological parents remains intact. This affects the personal status of the child in terms of ritual, inheritance and entering forbidden sexual relationships. Thus, information about the birth parents is important in Jewish adoptions. The Conservative rabbinate, in recognition of the intense familial bonds that develop within families having adopted children, considers adopted children to have the status of second-degree relatives, where the appropriate prohibitions against forbidden relationships apply.

Most of the halachic issues involving adoption are related to the personal status of the child and are dependent upon the status of the parents and the nature of their relationship. The simplest situation arises if the adopted child is non-Jewish. In these cases, conversion is necessary and the adoptive parents are henceforth considered to be the only parents (IM, *Yoreh Deah* #162; CJLS 04237; ARR #63). The adopted child's Hebrew name may even be referred to as son or daughter of the adoptive parents rather than of Abraham or Sarah, as is customary with adult converts (IM, *Yoreh Deah* #161; A. Reisner, 1988; ARR #63). Regardless of the status of the adoptive parents, though, the child assumes the ritual status of a *Yisrael* (Israelite) for the purposes of *pidyon haben* (redemption of the first born), being called to the Torah, marriage and divorce.

If the child is Jewish by birth, issues of personal status are more complicated. If both biological parents are known to be Jewish, no problem exists. The child retains the ritual status of the biological father, is considered the child of the biological father in terms of inheritance and a member of the genealogical family in terms of forbidden relationships. In the case where the mother is Jewish, but unmarried, the mother's statement about paternity is accepted. If she cannot establish paternity, then the child is presumed legitimate, since the mother's lineage is the critical factor (BT, *Kiddushin* 73a; MT, *Hilchot Issurei Bi'ah* 15:30, 31; Sh Ar, *Even HaEzer* 4:30,32). The concerns do focus, however, around the possibility of the child inadvertently entering into an incestuous or forbidden relationship with another Jew in the future. For example, if the adoptee has unknown siblings, then there is a slight chance that he or she could one day enter into an incestuous relationship with them. Or, if the child was the product of an adulterous or incestuous relationship, he or she is considered a *mamzer* (illegitimate) and ineligible to marry another Jew, except another *mamzer*. "A *mamzer* shall not enter the congregation of the Lord; even until the tenth generation, he shall not enter the congregation of the Lord" (*Deuteronomy* 23:3). If the parents are known to have been in such a situation, the child should be informed at some point.

In the event that the parentage is not known, the possibility that the child is a *mamzer* (*safek mamzer*) is raised in the Talmud (BT, *Kiddushin* 73a). These children fall into two categories, an *asufi* (a foundling where no information about either parent is available) or a *shetuki* (where the mother is unwilling to divulge the paternity). In the case of a possible *asufi*, the Talmud considers the child legitimate unless there is evidence that the child was totally unwanted and abandoned to die. For example, if the child was wrapped in a blanket, had a *brit milah* (ritual circumcision) or a *pidyon haben* (redemption of the first born), was left in a public place or near a synagogue where it would likely be found, it was not considered totally unwanted and, therefore, legitimate. The situation of a *shetuki* is more complex. When the mother is Jewish, the father is assumed to be the husband, and the child is legitimate. However, if the mother is unmarried, then there is the possibility that an incestuous relationship was involved. At the same time, there is a principle that the mother should be believed regarding the legitimacy of the child; a ruling by R. E. Landau in a similar case suggests that such a child is legitimate. In each of these circumstances, where the child is deemed Jewish (because the mother is Jewish) and not illegitimate, no conversion is necessary. In contrast to secular society, where all ties and relationships to the biological parents are severed, in Judaism, the personal status of the child remains forever linked to his or her biological lineage. That is, the child's status as a *Kohen, Levi* or *Yisrael* as well as his or her ability to enter into permitted relationships are determined by the biological and not the adoptive parents.

Adoption, therefore, remains a viable option for Jews struggling with infertility. Orthodox Jews may be more reticent adopting children of Jewish parents because of concerns regarding questions of personal status and the potential for their entering into forbidden relationships; however, there are no barriers toward adopting non-Jewish children. For Conservative and Reform Jews, the question of *mamzerut*, although recognized, has been deemed less critical because the statistical probability of an incestuous relationship occurring in the future is extremely small. The positive role toward adoption within the Jewish tradition exemplifies the centrality of children and family units to the future of the Jewish people, as well as the importance of maintaining links to the past.

**Infertility Treatment - Advanced Reproductive Technology**

The emotional, psychological and biological desire for human beings to have children is extremely strong. In Judaism, this is compounded by a positive religious mandate to "be fruitful and multiply" (*Genesis* 9:7). Unfortunately, infertility affects almost 20 percent of couples interested in having children, and only increases with age. The incidence of infertility, ironically, is likely to be higher among Jews, who often defer having families until they have completed their educations and established careers. Newer reproductive technologies represent significant advances in the treatment of infertility and provide options to overcome many of its causes.

The Torah introduces us to the pain of infertility in *Genesis* (17:15-22; 21:1-2; 25:21; 30:1). There, passages show Sarah, Rebecca and Rachel struggling with childlessness. Later in the Prophets (*Samuel* 1, 1:1-2:10), Hannah is shown desperately pleading with God for children. The Sages, appreciating how infertility strained the relationship between men, women and God, made these episodes a central theme of the readings from the Torah and Prophets on *Rosh Hashanah*, the Jewish New Year.

Infertility is usually diagnosed when a couple has been unable to conceive after one year of trying. Infertility may be traced to either the husband or the wife; up to 40 percent of infertility in couples is related to the male. Causes of male infertility include hormonal problems, azospermia (absence of sperm), oligospermia (insufficient sperm), abnormal sperm motility, defective semen, retrograde ejaculation, obstructed spermatic ducts, varicoceles and others. Among the causes of female infertility are hormonal abnormalities, defective or absent ovulation, anatomic deformities of the vagina, cervix, uterus, fallopian tubes or ovaries and abnormal cervical mucus. A thorough diagnostic evaluation of both partners, while necessary, raises halachic issues in the process.

Diagnosis of the husband involves testing for hormone levels, anatomic concerns related to the reproductive organs and their blood supply (such as obstructed ducts or a varicocele) and examination of the sperm and semen. There are no halachic concerns associated with obtaining blood for analysis or performing a thorough physical examination. However, procuring sperm for analysis poses difficulty because of the prohibition against *hash'hatat zera l'vatalah* ( the improper discharge or destruction of sperm "in vain") and possible interference with the normal sexual act (a violation of *onah*). Most authorities opine that because the ultimate goal here is procreation, harvesting sperm for analysis or artificial insemination does not violate the prohibition against discharge in vain (IM, *Even HaEzer* I #70, 71, II #16, 18, III #14, #27; NA, *Even HaEzer* 22:9; TE III #27, IX #51; ARR #153, 158; CARR #18). This leniency is based upon a discussion in the Talmud (BT, *Yebamot* 76a) in which a man who has suffered an injury to his penis is permitted to "emit seed" other than through intercourse in order to assess whether his injury has completely healed. Thus, the only remaining issue is interference with the sex act itself. Therefore, intercourse while subsequently harvesting the sperm from the vagina after ejaculation is the preferred halachic method in this situation (IM, *Even HaEzer* I #70, II #16, III #14, IV #27; NA, *Even HaEzer* 23:2). However, others have sanctioned collecting sperm after *coitus interruptus* or following intercourse using a condom (preferably with a perforation) or from an intravaginal receptacle (IM, *Even HaEzer* II #3; NA, *Even HaEzer* 23:2). Masturbation remains the least acceptable alternative because of the distinct rabbinic injunctions against it, particularly if it involves erotic stimulation (IM, *Even HaEzer* II #3; NA, *Even HaEzer* 23:2).[7] Direct aspiration or biopsy of the testes in order to procure sperm is occasionally utilized. Here too, opinions vary regarding its halachic acceptability, although Rabbis Feinstein and Waldenberg permit it as a last resort (IM, *Even HaEzer* II #3, TE IX #51). R. Waldenberg is generally in

---

7. Rabbi Elliot Dorff informs me that he is definitely *not* against masturbation for the procurement of sperm as an assisted reproductive technique "because the act is definitely not intended to waste the seed but rather to use it for its intended purpose. Some Orthodox rabbis agree with me on this. Moreover, gynecologists have told me that collecting the sperm from the woman's vaginal cavity after intercourse is simply not practical." See *Matters of Life and Death*, p.52.

agreement with this overall approach to male infertility (TE VII #48:1:7, IX #51:1, XI #42:8, XVI #41:2, XX #48, XXI #36).

The problems encountered in the evaluation of the wife center around the issue of *niddah*. *Niddah* is the state of ritual impurity that affects a woman when menstrual blood from the uterus is present in the vagina. (The term for the presence of uterine blood in the vagina during times other than at menstruation is *zavah*, although *niddah* and *zavah* will be treated identically in this discussion). From the time a woman becomes a *niddah,* she is prohibited according to *halacha* from having physical contact or sexual relations with her husband until after she has experienced seven consecutive days in which no vaginal blood can be detected and has properly immersed herself in the *mikvah* (ritual bath). In order for a woman to become a *niddah*, the blood must naturally originate in the uterus. Thus, blood that is caused by a wound or injury (*makkah*) does not technically result in a woman becoming a *niddah*. Unfortunately, because it is usually impossible to determine whether a wound is present or precisely where the blood originated, it is presumed that the blood is of uterine origin, rendering the woman a *niddah*. The diagnostic evaluation of women for infertility involves numerous procedures (physical exam, cannulation and visualization of the vagina, cervix, uterus and fallopian tubes, post-coital cervical mucus sampling, dilatation and uterine biopsy, hystosalpingogram and laparoscopy), some of which may cause mild bleeding. Thus, knowledge and careful attention to the details involved will allow differentiation between situations in which the woman is a *niddah* and in which she is not. This is critical, since numerous aspects of the evaluation and treatment of the couple require intimate contact, which is halachically prohibited when the wife is a *niddah*.

In principle, most halachic authorities sanction the use of reproductive techniques as an option for infertile married couples. In practice, however, concerns are raised by the potential outcome of some of these methods, such as adultery, the permissibility for future relations between the couple, the possible need for divorce, issues of paternity and maternity, illegitimacy of the children (*mamzerut*), requirements for child support, inheritance, fulfillment of ritual roles (such as for *Kohanim*), the potential for later incest or forbidden marriage, the prohibition against the destruction of seed in vain and the exposure of women to unnecessary danger. These issues will be highlighted in a discussion of the different methods involved.

Among the oldest available techniques are Artificial Insemination with Husband as Donor (AIH) and Artificial Insemination with Anonymous Donor Sperm (AID). These methods, although not as successful as newer modifications in all circumstances, are best suited for cases of male infertility or where there is a physical barrier to the passage of sperm. AIH is a technique in which the husband's sperm is collected and then implanted, usually by injection into the uterus (intrauterine insemination), where fertilization occurs. This method is generally considered to be the most acceptable according to *halacha* (IM, *Even HaEzer* I #10, II #18; Auerbach, Noam, 1968; CJLS 042649, 061949, 012052, 022378; ARR #157). A minority of decisors (R. Waldenberg) believe that AIH is morally unacceptable, although not technically in violation of *halacha*. The main legal objection to AIH relates to the method of procuring the husband's sperm because of the injunction against *hashchatat zera l'vatalah* and the possibility of violating *onah*. The same hierarchy of techniques used for the procurement of sperm for infertility analysis applies to this technique: post-coital sperm harvesting is the preferred method, followed by the use of a condom during intercourse, *coitus interruptus* and masturbation. All Orthodox authorities are strict in forbidding the mixture of the husband's sperm with that of others to enhance its potency (IM, *Even HaEzer* I #10; TE, IX, 51:4, XIII, #93, XV # 45; R. Auerbach, R. Noam, 1958). Both Rabbis Feinstein and Auerbach have permitted compromises by allowing sexual contact during a woman's *niddah* period if necessary for fertilization (IM, *Even HaEzer* II #18, *Yoreh Deah* II #84; Auerbach, Noam, 1958).

A related subject involves sperm banking in anticipation of infertility. Men afflicted with diseases such as cancer, which, through treatment by surgery, chemotherapy or radiation, will result in sterility may want to donate sperm for the purpose of future artificial insemination. Frozen sperm may be stored for prolonged periods of time and still achieve fertilization with a reasonable degree of success. Although most Orthodox authorities permit this practice since the purpose is aimed at the fulfillment of the *mitzvah* of procreation, some advocate restraint (NA IV, *Even HaEzer* 23:1) or limit it to married men (R. Bakshi-Doron).

AID involves the use of sperm from an unknown donor to achieve fertilization of the wife's egg *in utero*. The use of donor sperm (or eggs) raises considerable ethical concerns in both secular and religious communities. Among the arguments that have been raised against the use of donor gametes are: (1) the procedure dissociates procreation exclusively through marriage; (2) it compromises the genealogy of the resulting child; (3) it may encourage adultery; (4) it has similarities to eugenics; and (5) it stigmatizes sterility by suggesting that it could legitimately threaten the marital bond. These moral questions are shared by the rabbinic authorities involved in the evaluation of AID.

Halachically, Orthodox authorities uniformly consider AID using a Jewish donor unacceptable for several reasons. First, since the *mitzvah* of procreation is incumbent on the husband and not the wife, the question arises as to whether having children through AID fulfills that commandment since the husband is not the source of the sperm. Second, there is disagreement about whether or not AID constitutes adultery. The Biblical prohibition against adultery states: "and with the wife of your neighbor you shall not lie carnally to defile yourself with her" (*Leviticus* 18:20). Many [R. Auerbach (Noam 1958), R. Feinstein (IM, *Even HaEzer*

I #10) and R. Waldenberg (TE, III #24)] argue that adultery requires the performance of an actual sexual act, while others state that even the presence of another man's semen in a married woman's vagina is tantamount to that (R. Y. Teitelbaum). If AID does constitute adultery, then the children are classified as illegitimate (*mamzerim*) and the couple is subsequently prohibited from cohabiting. Rabbis Feinstein (IM, *Even HaEzer* I #10) and Auerbach (Noam 1958) consider such a child of such a union to be legitimate, while R. Waldenberg considers the offspring to be of questionable status (*safek mamzer)* (TE, III #24). Other concerns associated with AID using a Jewish donor include the potential for incest and forbidden marriage between children of a common Jewish father and concerns resulting from the paternity of the child since halachically, the genetic father is considered the father. The issue of paternity affects the inheritance of the child, even though the husband has raised and supported the child since gestation. The status of the child vis-à-vis roles in Jewish ritual (*Kohen* or *Levi*) are also assigned according to the biological father. Because of the many complexities involved, even Rabbis Auerbach and Feinstein, who were generally lenient in permitting the use of reproductive technologies, prohibited AID using a

Jewish donor. R. Waldenberg forbids AID and considers it to be morally unacceptable (TE, IX #51:4). Furthermore, all halachic authorities prohibit a Jewish man from donating sperm to be used for artificial insemination with any women other than his wife. The CJLS, in earlier decisions, forbade artificial insemination by a man other than the husband (CJLS 042649, 061949, 012052, 022378) and related Reform responsa displayed caution (ARR #158). More recently, Conservative (R. Dorff) and Reform (ARR #157; CARR #19) authorities have sanctioned AID using a Jewish donor. Their reasoning is based upon the fact that no adulterous relationship occurred because there was no act of sexual intercourse and the chances of the offspring having an incestuous relationship are extremely small, especially if careful birth records are kept and the information is made available to the child. Orthodox authorities such as Rabbis Auerbach (Noam 1958) and Feinstein (IM, *Even HaEzer* IV #71), have held that AID may be permissible under extreme circumstances if the donor is a non-Jew, although R. Waldenberg (TE, IX #51:4) is opposed to AID altogether. A non-Jew as the donor obviates many, but not all, of the halachic problems related to the personal status of the child that arise when the donor is Jewish. For example, the child, even though "adopted" and raised by the biological mother's husband, is not halachically his offspring (TE, IX #51), and is therefore not entitled to the benefits of inheritance, unless specifically superseded by a will. Another issue relates to the ritual status of the child, who, according to R. Auerbach, assumes the status of the mother as a *Kohen*, *Levi* or *Yisrael*. Such a situation may lead to public embarrassment of the child or father, and must be considered when counseling couples regarding AID. Auerbach also ruled that a first-born son requires redemption (*pidyon haben*) as usual (NA, *Even HaEzer* 1:2). Finally, all Orthodox authorities require the husband's consent in order for the wife to undergo AID. Failure to obtain his permission has been considered legitimate grounds for divorce and authorization for the procedure obligates the husband to provide financial support for the child (IM, *Even HaEzer* I #10; TE IX #51:4).

At present, the use of techniques involving variations of In Vitro (test-tube) Fertilization (IVF) are becoming more common. Eggs are harvested from the wife and then mixed with sperm in the laboratory. If conception is allowed to occur and the embryos are transferred to the uterus, the procedure is known as In Vitro

Fertilization with Embryo Transfer (ET). A more refined procedure involves combining the eggs and sperm and transferring and instilling the mixture into the fallopian tube, called Gamete Intra-Fallopian Transfer (GIFT). If fertilization occurs and the formed embryos are, in turn, placed into the fallopian tube, the procedure is known as Zygote Intra-Fallopian Transfer (ZIFT).

Most Orthodox and all Conservative and Reform authorities rule that IVF using the husband's sperm is permissible. All of the caveats concerning the appropriateness of various techniques for procurement of the husband's sperm apply and no other sperm donors may be used. If the donor cannot be the husband, Orthodox decisors prefer for the donor to be a non-Jew in order to avoid the issues of personal status, forbidden relationships and adultery. Conservative and Reform authorities are less concerned with these issues since the possibility of such an offspring marrying an unknown relative in the future is extremely remote. Those Orthodox authorities who consider AID an act of adultery are more lenient regarding IVF-ET, GIFT and ZIFT from another donor because the sperm is placed in the uterus rather than the vagina. In each of these cases, the child is regarded as Jewish by all since the mother is Jewish.

The use of donor ova is potentially more problematic, particularly as it relates to the establishment of maternity. Halachic opinions differ over whether the gestational or genetic mother is authentic, or if there is actually dual motherhood. The determination of maternity will affect the religious status of the child and impacts on the need for conversion. Another concern relates to the donor subjecting herself to an unnecessary risk. Because the procedures and techniques involved are common and safe, they are permitted ["the multitude has trodden upon them" (BT, *Shabbat* 129b)]. However, some authorities recommend ultrasound-guided harvesting of ova over laparoscopic harvesting because it avoids anesthesia and surgery (Halperin). Since the woman is not required to bear children, she cannot be compelled to undergo such a procedure as no one is obligated (or perhaps even permitted) to expose themselves to risk in order to fulfill a positive commandment (IM, *Even HaEzer* III #12; R. Bleich).

Additional issues involved with advanced reproductive technologies include the use of gametes donated by relatives, the fate of the remaining unimplanted embryos, the unknown potential for genetic abnormalities in the offspring, sex determination or selection, and the role of fetal reductive surgery in the event of a multiple pregnancy. All Orthodox halachic authorities prohibit the use of gametes from relatives, reasoning that sexual contact between relatives that is considered incestuous and expressly forbidden by the Torah is still forbidden if done artificially. This analysis is similar to that used in forbidding AID using a Jewish donor. However, Conservative (R. Dorff) and Reform (CARR #19) authorities have taken a more lenient view based upon the notion that since no sexual act occurs, there is no adulterous relationship -- a situation that is no different from that involving AID.

Although the fate of unutilized frozen embryos in society at large is controversial, the halachic position regarding their disposal is clear. Unimplanted fertilized eggs are not considered embryos and therefore have no legal standing. Their destruction is considered neither abortion nor murder (R. C.D. HaLevy, R. M. Eliyahu, R. Bleich). In a related matter, authorities from each branch of Judaism (Waldenberg, Bleich, Dorff, Jacob) have suggested that it may be permissible to use aborted fetal tissue and unutilized embryos for the purposes of scientific research.

Since a fetus is not a person in the full legal sense of the term, the requirements for burial and prohibitions against deriving benefit from the dead do not apply. Based upon the complex circumstances and issues involved with the use of advanced reproductive techniques, a hierarchy can be established based upon the opinions published -

| **Rank** (1=most preferred) | **Method of Sperm Procurement*** |
|---|---|
| 1 | Intercourse followed by vaginal harvesting of sperm |
| 2 | Intercourse using intravaginal receptacle |
| 3 | Intercourse using perforated condom |
| 4 | Intercourse using nonperforated condom |
| 5 | *Coitus interruptus* |
| 6 | Masturbation |

| **Rank** | **Method of Assisted Reproduction*** |
|---|---|
| 1 | Artificial Insemination with Husband's Sperm |
| 2 | Gamete Intra-Fallopian Transfer with Husband's Sperm (GIFT-H) |
| 3 | In-Vitro Fertilization w/ Husband's Sperm + Zygote/Embryo Transfer (ZIFT-H) |
| 4 | In-Vitro w/ Non-Jewish Donor Sperm + Zygote/Embryo Transfer (ZIFT-D) |
| 5 | Gamete Intra-Fallopian Transfer with Non-Jewish Donor Sperm (GIFT-D) |
| 6 | Artificial Insemination with Non-Jewish Donor Sperm (AID) |

7 In-Vitro Fertilization with Non-Jewish Donor Ova + Embryo Transfer (ZIFT-Do)

8 In-Vitro Fertilization with Jewish Donor Ova + Embryo Transfer (ZIFT-JDo)

* = Not all methods are endorsed by all authorities

The desire for children is so strong for many couples that it behooves halachic decisors to carefully evaluate all of these new technologies to maximize their availability to Jewish families. This will help alleviate some of their pain while, in turn, strengthen the Jewish community. Sanctioning the use of these methods exemplifies the sensitivity of Jewish law to the frailties of the human condition.

## Infertility Treatment - Surrogate Motherhood

Few issues in recent years have engendered as much ethical debate in the public sector as that of surrogate motherhood, pitting the rights of the biological parents against those of the host mother -- and both, at times, against the best interests of the child. This interest has affected the Jewish community as well, as the halachic quandries posed by the use of surrogate gestational mothers are no less complex than those within the secular sphere.

The use of a surrogate facilitates the treatment of two forms of female infertility. The first type involves a woman who is incapable of producing viable ova. In such a case, the egg may be supplied by the "surrogate," in which case fertilization is accomplished by artificial insemination and the surrogate carries the fetus to term. Alternatively, the egg can be obtained from another source, in which case fertilization is accomplished using in vitro techniques with the resultant embryo transferred to the surrogate, who carries the fetus to term. The second form of infertility involves a female who produces viable eggs but cannot carry a pregnancy to term. In this instance, conception either occurs naturally and the embryo is then harvested and transferred to the surrogate, or ova are harvested from the woman and fertilized in vitro with the husband's sperm and then the embryo is transferred to the surrogate, who provides the "gestational incubator." In each of these cases, the husband donates the sperm; in neither instance does a sexual act involving the surrogate take place.

Surrogate motherhood has posed numerous moral and legal complications in the civil and religious arenas. Among the most difficult issues confronting society are the rights of the biological parents versus those of the birth mother. A number of Orthodox authorities (Rabbis Auerbach and Waldenberg) are opposed to the use of surrogates, although the practice has recently been sanctioned by the Israeli courts (Israeli Surrogacy Law, 1996). In addition, Rabbi A. Rosenfeld has argued that acting as a host would be halachically permissible since a married woman is permitted to act as a wet nurse for another couple's child (Sh Ar, *Even HaEzer* 80:14; *Ar HaSh*, *Even HaEzer* 13:24) and Rabbis E.D. Clark and Z. Silverman have suggested that surrogacy would be halachically acceptable in cases of high risk pregnancy. The Conservative and Reform rabbinates have also given their approval (D. Lincoln, 1998, A. Mackler, 1998; CARR #18; ARR #159). Those justifying surrogacy point to the precedent set by the handmaidens in the Torah who bore children for the infertile matriarchs Sarah and Rachel. Conservative and Reform opinions employ the rationale that use of all available reproductive technologies to alleviate the problem of infertility helps obviate the problem of a declining Jewish birthrate. Nevertheless, Jewish law raises numerous additional questions over issues such as the establishment of maternity and paternity, adultery, the legitimacy of the children, the personal status of the offspring with respect to religious duties and inheritance, the potential for incest or forbidden marriage and the exposure of the surrogate mother to unnecessary danger.

Determining maternity in Jewish law is particularly controversial and hinges on the timing of when a maternal-child relationship is established. Is maternity established at the moment of fertilization or at the time of parturition? If it is at the time of conception (fertilization), the egg donor is considered the mother, which obviates other problems, such as the need for conversion of the child to Judaism, matters of inheritance, and the child's personal status. If maternity is established at birth, however, the surrogate is considered the legal mother.

The question of maternity is further complicated in cases where there is embryo transfer from the genetic mother to the surrogate. The Talmud (BT, *Yebamot* 69b) considers a fetus "merely water" (*maya d'alma*) for the first 40 days of gestation. Therefore, if the embryo is transferred prior to that, and maternity is determined at birth, then the surrogate is considered the mother. If the embryo is transferred after 40 days, then the removal of the embryo from the genetic mother could be considered as a "birth" because the Talmud states that formation is complete at that time. In that case, the embryo donor would be the mother. If maternity is established at fertilization, however, then the genetic mother is always the mother.

Most authorities consider maternity to be established at birth. Therefore, the surrogate is legally the mother according to *halacha* and the child's personal status is to be determined based upon that. All authorities agree that the child of a non-Jewish surrogate is not Jewish according to *halacha* and needs to convert (NA, *Even HaEzer* 5:2; CJLS 1985; Rabbis D. Lincoln, 1985; E. Spitz ,1997; A. Mackler, 1997). This conclusion is based upon the fact that if a pregnant woman converts to Judaism, the child is considered hers and her first-born son must be redeemed (a ceremony known as *pidyon haben*) even though he was not Jewish at the time of conception (JT, *Yebamot* 11:2). R. Auerbach, although opposed to surrogate motherhood, considered both the genetic mother and the surrogate to be mothers and required conversion of the child if neither was Jewish (NA, *Even HaEzer* 5:2). Similar arguments for dual maternity have been advanced by R. Bleich (Orthodox) and R. E. Spitz (Conservative, 1996).

The argument for two mothers implies that a maternal-child relationship can be recognized both at the time of conception and at birth. The rationale for maternity being established at conception is based upon the Talmudic view that ensoulment occurs at conception (BT, *Sanhedrin* 91b) and the fact that the child of a pregnant proselyte is also considered a proselyte (BT, Yebamot78a). Because no actual sexual contact occurs between the husband/father and the surrogate, there is no adulterous relationship and the child is considered legitimate. A Reform responsum by R. Jacob (ARR #159) permits the use of a married surrogate, and Rosenfeld concurs that a married woman may serve in this capacity, but is required to separate from her husband for 90 days to ensure the child's paternity (Sh Ar, *Even HaEzer* 13:6). As with artificial insemination using donor sperm, most Orthodox authorities, concerned with the possibility of future incestuous relationships, are opposed to the use of Jewish surrogates. There is no question of paternity, which clearly resides with the biological father. Most authorities also hold that the father has fulfilled his procreative obligation under these circumstances.

There are concerns related to the role of the surrogate in this process. In terms of assuming physical risk in undertaking such a pregnancy, it would seem that this would be permitted if she were in good health based upon the concept that "the multitude has trodden upon them" (BT, *Shabbat* 129b). The contract with the surrogate poses certain problems according to Jewish law. Contrary to American civil law, which considers the sale of children to be illegal, R. Bleich points out that Jewish law does not consider it as such. However, he raises the issue that the contract is invalid and hence unenforceable because it is executed before the surrogate is inseminated. Thus, according to *halacha*, should the gestational mother decide to keep the child, she would be legally entitled and the father would be morally and financially responsible for its upbringing. Whether the resolution of this dilemma falls under the rubric of *dina d'malchuta dina* is unclear at this time.

The use of surrogate hosts to remedy infertility poses several unique halachic problems in addition to societal issues. Many of these dilemmas have no definitive answers and serve to demonstrate that as future developments occur, halachic precedents and solutions may become increasingly more difficult to devise.

## Infertility Treatment – Cloning

Cloning is the creation of a genetically identical replica of a given entity. That is, the clone is a perfect copy having the identical genetic composition (genotype) and physical appearance (phenotype) of the original. The scientific methodology to clone plants and lower forms of life has been available for some time; it is only recently that scientists have reported successfully cloning adult mammals. Ethical discussions about cloning have been initiated because of the tremendous potential for this new technology to have an impact on a host of therapeutic modalities and concerns about the possibility of eventually cloning an entire human being.

Numerous potential uses of human cloning technology exist that could radically alter the current practice of medicine. Cloning could be employed to eliminate the transmission of genetic diseases from parents to offspring by correcting them and subsequently using the corrected cells for reproduction. In the area of infertility treatment, cloning could allow people who were otherwise incapable of producing viable sperm or ova to conceive children. This technology could also be used in cancer treatment and tissue regeneration. Among the more novel and exciting uses of cloning would be the development of genetically engineered "replacement parts," human organs that were maintained in animal hosts that could be used for organ transplantation or specific cell types that could be implanted in people with degenerative conditions.

Yet along with the potential benefits of cloning, there are uncharted areas that raise moral dilemmas. The long-term viability of cloned cells, organs or organisms is unknown, as is the potential for medical problems that have not yet been anticipated. Moreover, concerns have been voiced about the advisability of creating a situation in which the processes of aging and death would be dramatically altered. One can envision that aging would be accompanied by a successive series of organ or cell replacement therapies to ward off death for as long as possible. People could stockpile their cells so that they could clone themselves and return to life after death. These ethical concerns have led to the call for a moratorium on any attempts to clone humans. In addition to these societal ramifications, many unique halachic questions arise related to the use of cloning. For example, are human clones considered human beings? If so, who are the parents, and have they fulfilled the *mitzvah* of procreation? What are clones' relationship to siblings? Are they to be considered Jewish? How is the personal religious status of the clone determined, and what religious obligations do they have?

The most compelling argument in support of cloning is that it enhances our ability to fulfill the obligation "heal you shall heal" (*Exodus* 21:19). This phrase, coupled with the earlier blessing to "...be fruitful and multiply; fill the earth and subdue it, ...." (*Genesis* 1:28) provides permission to develop and employ such potentially beneficial technology. In certain situations, such as treatment of infertility, cloning might be halachically more advantageous than artificial insemination and in vitro fertilization since the concerns associated with procurement of sperm and *hashchatat zera l'vatalah* would be eliminated. However, there are also halachic considerations that bode against cloning. Based upon the biblical commentary of Nachmanides (*Leviticus* 19:19), cloning could be considered to violate *derech hateva* (the way of nature), which is a direct affront to God and the Divine scheme. Human cloning, an essentially asexual process that may not even involve contributions from both sexes, represents an encroachment on the normal process of procreation that is beyond the pale. Use of human cloning to create genetically superior people (eugenics), might also violate prohibitions against certain mixtures of species (*kilayim*).

In terms of the humanity of a clone, the only example to draw upon in rabbinic literature is that of the mythical *golem* (an anthropoid created from dust). There are several different opinions regarding the status of a *golem*: an animal, a human, a human if it can speak, and not a living creature. However, since a clone differs from a *golem* in that it is derived from humans, not dust, and is born after gestation, R. Bleich suggests that it would be considered human. Different problems would arise if gestation and birth occurred through other species. Issues involving the religious and personal status of a clone have not been resolved, and possibilities abound. For example, in the case of a mother cloning herself, the clone would have no halachic father; perhaps the mother could be that father. Such an arrangement has a tremendous impact on matters of inheritance and the permissibility of future marriages, among other issues. These issues will have to await clarification as the technology evolves.

*Eight months later. Devorah undergoes artificial insemination with Gabriel as the donor and eventually conceives. An ultrasound examination early in the pregnancy suggests that there may be four fetuses. Devorah's obstetrician feels that it will be too risky for her to try to carry all of them to term and suggests aborting two or three. Although Devorah would never consider abortion under normal circumstances, she accepts the doctor's advice while trying not to let the pain she feels about aborting these fetuses interfere with the joy she feels from carrying her own baby. She is beginning to believe that things are finally starting to "go her way." The couple is interested in having an amniocentesis performed and trying to select a boy and a girl.*

Since antiquity, potential parents -- influenced by cultural and economic factors -- have been intrigued with the notion of choosing or determining the sex of their children.

**Issues**: Sex preference and selection

**Sex Preference and Selection**

There are aspects of Jewish tradition that promote, although perhaps inadvertently, the desire to preselect the sex of one's children. Men are obligated to perform more *mitzvot* than women and have traditionally enjoyed a more prominent role in Jewish ritual, communal and economic life. Women have been held in greater esteem with regard to family and have been charged with the primary responsibility for the religious atmosphere of the home and for Jewish continuity. (According to *halacha*, Jewishness is solely determined by the religion of the mother). Further, the laws of inheritance give preference to male offspring, although the Torah acknowledges a place for women, as seen in the story of the daughters of Zelophehad (*Numbers* 27:1-11). Nevertheless, these practical considerations can lead potential parents to preferring that their unborn child be one sex and not the other.

The Sages were fascinated with the idea of sex determination. The Talmud (BT, *Niddah* 31a,b) states: "If the woman emits her semen first, she bears a male child; if a man emits his semen first, she bears a female child; for it is said: 'If a woman emits semen and bears a man child'" (*Leviticus* 12:2). Numerous commentators, including Rashi, Ibn Ezra, Malbim, Sforno and Nachmanides, interpret this to mean that if the woman reaches orgasm first, the child will be male. Rashi even suggests having intercourse twice in a row to ensure this because the male has a prolonged refractory period. Numerous Talmudic sources advocate various methodologies for male sex selection. R.Yitzchak (BT, *B'rachot* 5b) suggests orienting the bed in a north-south direction; Rabbis Eliezer and Yehoshua (BT, *Bava Batra* 10b) advocate giving *tzedakah* (charity) and charming one's wife so that she is positively predisposed to the performance of the *mitzvah* of procreation; and R. Yochanon (*Shevuot*18b) posits that abstaining from sex immediately prior to menstruation will yield a male child. Despite the enthusiasm for such manipulation, the fallibility of these methods was recognized: "Did not many ...act in this manner yet it did not avail them?" (BT, *Niddah* 71a).

Modern medicine has developed several methods of determining the sex of a child, both before and after intercourse. The pre-coital method involves sperm procurement followed by separation of androsperm (male) and gynosperm (female), as is used in artificial insemination, after which the selected sperm are inserted into the female. Although the success rate of this method is 75-95 percent, the chance of successful fertilization is decreased in comparison to the use of unmanipulated sperm. The timing of intercourse can affect the sex of the child, with the proportion of male births highest if sex occurs immediately before ovulation. This may be halachically problematic, though, as a woman may still be a *niddah* at that point in her cycle. Finally, manipulation of the pH of vaginal and cervical fluid can influence the sex of the offspring, since an alkaline pH favors male sperm. The post-coital methods are considerably more invasive and technically challenging. Chromosomal analysis of in-vitro fertilized embryos or amniotic fluid obtained through amniocentesis can reliably determinate the sex of the child. However, these methods are associated with greater risk to the mother along with increased cost and, therefore, have not been widely endorsed by the medical community as a preferred method for sex selection.

It is apparent from the foregoing discussion that the concept of sex selection is not halachically forbidden. Acceptable methods would include those that did not interfere with the requirements of *onah*, violate the ban against *hashchatat zera l'vatalah* (the improper discharge or destruction of sperm) or conflict with the laws of *niddah* (ritual impurity). However, serious concerns have been raised by Orthodox (R. Bleich, Rosner), Conservative and Reform (R. Schiff) leaders regarding the social and demographic consequences of such technology with respect to the future population needs of the Jewish people. Since Jews have had below average birth rates for several decades, there is a fear that the ready availability of sex selection will further contribute to this negative trend. Other reservations include the potential erosion of marital intimacy. Similarly, utilization of any of the halachically acceptable methods of sex selection would also be prohibited if the results would lead to abortion. The question of preselecting the sex of a child by a couple having in vitro fertilization, in which some of the fertilized eggs are not going to be implanted anyway, is controversial. In general, the prevailing opinion among Orthodox and Conservative authorities is that sex selection in this situation is not permitted, as the primary goal is the treatment of infertility by as natural a process as possible; sex selection is inconsistent with this purpose. Reform authorities (ARR #160; Schiff), while still raising questions, have been more somewhat more lenient in this regard.[8]

When information about the sex of the child will have an impact on its future health, permission for preselection has been more forthcoming. For example, Rabbi Auerbach prohibited sperm separation for the purpose of sex selection under normal circumstances, but allowed it to prevent transmission of sex-linked hereditary diseases such as hemophilia (NA, *Even HaEzer* 1:1).

The prohibition against sex selection in certain circumstances represents an example of *halacha* placing limits on the use of modern technology. Not everything that can be done ought to be done.

---

8. Conservative Rabbi Elliot Dorff argues that "a more urgent consideration, it seems to me, is that the command to procreate is understood by Jewish law to require both a boy and a girl, and if you have begotten, say, four or five children of only one gender, you may want to make sure that the next one fulfills the commandment. Although I am in general against sex selection, and although I would interpret Jewish law in our day to say that fulfilling the commandment requires minimally two children of whatever gender (see my *Matters of Life and Death*, p.44), if a couple wanted to fulfill the commandment as it has been traditionally interpreted, or if they simply want to have at least one child of the other gender, I would allow the use of measures to insure a child of the other gender in such circumstances."

## Multi-Gestational Pregnancy Reduction

A frequent by-product of infertility therapy using hormonal manipulation or advanced reproductive technologies is multi-gestational pregnancy, which is associated with increased risk to the mother and fetuses. These mothers have a greater incidence of prenatal and perinatal complications. The threat of pre-eclampsia (hypertension, kidney problems and seizures) exceeds 20 percent and that of postpartum hemorrhage, 35 percent. Fetal mortality is increased in direct proportion to the number of fetuses: 16 percent for triplets, 21 percent for quadruplets or quintuplets and 40 percent for sextuplets. For these reasons, pregnancy reduction is often recommended for women with multiple pregnancies.

Judaism forbids the sacrifice of one human being to save another. The Talmud (JT, *Terumot* 8:12) discusses a situation where heathens said to a group of Jewish women: "Surrender one of you to us so that we may defile her, or else we will defile you all." The Talmud rules that all should suffer defilement rather than surrender a single woman. Maimonides agrees (MT *Yesodei HaTorah* 5:5). An exception to this rule is the case of a *rodef* (pursuer), when it is permissible to sacrifice a life in order to defend oneself. In the case of a pregnant woman who is carrying multiple fetuses at high risk for complications, similar reasoning can be applied and a case made for therapeutic abortion. The fetuses are considered potential threats to her life and, therefore, one or more can be sacrificed. Pregnancy reduction might also be sanctioned if the birth of multiple children results in significant psychological or emotional strain on the mother.

When examined from the perspective of the best interests of the fetus, the issue becomes more complicated. Since the fetus is not considered a complete human being until birth, the overriding consideration is the health and well-being of the mother (see previous discussion of abortion). In the absence of any increased risk to the mother, is there any halachic justification for fetal reduction? Several opinions have been advanced. One approach is based upon the idea that some of the fetuses could be considered pursuers (*rodfim*) of the others. An exception to the Talmudic dictum discussed previously is that if it is clear that all threatened must die, then some authorities have permitted a few to be sacrificed if chosen at random or by lottery so that the others might live. Similarly, according to R. Auerbach, if all of the fetuses are destined to die, then the same reasoning can be applied

(NA, *Choshen Mishpat* 425:1:25). Other Orthodox authorities (Rabbis C.D. HaLevy, M. Eliyahu) have taken a more lenient approach, permitting pregnancy reduction based on the fact that a significant number of the fetuses will likely be born with severe mental or physical disabilities. As noted by R. Dorff, Conservative and Reform rabbis would undoubtedly agree with this more lenient view.

In practice, since multi-gestational pregnancies are associated with significantly increased maternal risk, this usually provides sufficient justification for pregnancy reduction. As with abortion, because the embryo is considered "mere fluid" before the 40th day of gestation, many authorities are liberal about abortion during this time, others permit it freely, and a minority of rabbis do not allow it at all. Thus, although pregnancy reduction can be performed at any stage during pregnancy, it should preferentially be done before 40 days post-conception.

Pregnancy reduction undertaken for the health of the mother or the fetuses provides another example of *halacha*'s value of existing life over potential life.

*Two of the fetuses are successfully aborted at random and the pregnancy continues. However, in the fourth month, Devorah is admitted to the hospital with signs of toxemia of pregnancy (hypertension, renal dysfunction, glucose intolerance). The doctors are worried that she could lose her transplanted kidney and pancreas and recommend that the pregnancy be terminated. At first, Devorah refuses to submit to an abortion. Gabriel, her parents, in-laws, siblings and physicians try in vain to convince her. Gabriel is devastated and tries to convince Devorah that he cannot go on living without her.*

Abortion has been one of the most controversial issues in American politics during the past two decades since its legalization (Roe v. Wade, 1974). The debate over abortion has influenced political campaigns and elections at all levels and led to protests, bombings and murders.

**Issue:** Abortion

## Abortion

In Jewish law, abortion is generally prohibited for several reasons. Judaism sanctifies life. Man and woman were the only life forms individually created by God; all other species were created in total. This teaches us that it was worthwhile for God to have created the entire world for one individual. A similar thought is related in the Talmud (BT, *Sanhedrin* 37a): "One who saves a single life is (viewed) as though (s)he has saved an entire world. One who destroys a life is as if (s)he destroyed an entire world." One of the Seven Noahide Laws can also be interpreted as referring to abortion: "Whoever sheds the blood of man in man, his blood shall be shed, for in the image of God He made man." (*Genesis* 9:6). The Talmud (BT, *Sanhedrin* 57b) asks: "Who is man in man?" R. Yishmael interprets this to mean a fetus. The Rabbis deduce from this that a gentile is prohibited from murdering anyone, even a fetus.

Although the subject of abortion is not directly discussed in the Torah, the issue of feticide is addressed (*Exodus* 21:22-23), which provides guidance for subsequent Talmudic discussions regarding abortion: "When two men fight, and one of them pushes a pregnant woman and miscarriage results, and no other misfortune, the one responsible shall be fined as the woman's husband may ask him, the payment based on the reckoning of the judges. But if any harm [to the mother] ensues, you shall give life for life..." From these verses, it is clear that feticide is prohibited and condemned, although not considered murder. The penalty imposed for causing the death of a fetus is only monetary, while the punishment for murdering a human being (the mother) is death, suggesting that the value accorded to a fetus is lesser than that of a person. This is supported by the fact that the fetus is referred to by the term *yeladeha* (her fetus), as opposed to *nefesh* (soul), which the Torah uses to denote life (as in *Exodus* 21:23, which describes the death of a man, and in *Genesis* 2:7, which describes the blowing of the soul of life into humankind). For these reasons, abortion is not technically considered murder or manslaughter since the fetus is not considered a whole person until it emerges from the mother's body (BT, Sandedrin 84b).

Jewish law recognizes several statuses of the fetus during pregnancy. Rashi considers the fetus a limb of the mother (*uber yerech imo*) throughout pregnancy. In his classification, the fetus may be considered alive, as are all cells or organs of a larger entity, but it is only a "potential life" until it is born. According to the Talmud (BT, *Yebamot* 69b), an embryo is believed to be "mere water" (*maya d'alma*). This interpretation is based on the length of time that the daughter of a *Kohen* that became widowed had to wait before she could eat sanctified food with her family in the event she were pregnant. If she was less than 40 days pregnant, she was not considered ritually impure and was able to eat with her family. After 40 days, the fetus acquired greater status, so she could not eat with her family. For example, during Temple times, if a woman spontaneously aborted after 40 days, she was required to bring a sacrifice as though she had delivered a live baby. This supports the notion that a fetus over 40 days' gestation has a legal status more akin to that of a "person."

Abortions are permitted according to *halacha* under a variety of circumstances, but there is no unanimity of rabbinic opinion. An abortion is generally allowed, or even mandated, when the mother's life is at risk, a situation requiring *pikuach nefesh*. In the classic text on this subject, the Mishnah (*Ohalot* 7:6) states: "If a woman is undergoing a perilous pregnancy, the fetus must be dismembered limb by limb and removed because her life takes precedence over its life. If the greater portion of the fetus has been delivered, it must not be touched because one life must not be sacrificed for another." The Talmud (BT, *Sanhedrin* 72b) elaborates on this as follows: "If the head has emerged, it may not be harmed because one life (*nefesh*) is not sacrificed for the sake of another. Is the fetus not a pursuer (*rodef*)? The case is different because [the mother] is being pursued by heaven."

Rashi interprets these statements as follows: "Until the child has emerged into the world, it is not considered a person and it is permissible to destroy it in order to save the mother's life. However, once the head has emerged, it is considered as though it was born, and one may not harm it because it is forbidden to take one life for another." Thus, according to Rashi, the fetus, as a non-person, has a lower status than the mother until its head emerges during the birth process, and its life is subordinate to the mother's.

Maimonides (MT, *Hilchot Rotzeach* 1:9) takes a more stringent view and considers the fetus under such circumstances to be a potential murderer (*rodef*), threatening the life of the mother:

> "There is also a negative commandment to have no mercy toward a pursuer (*rodef*). Thus, the Sages taught that if a woman has difficulty in childbirth, the fetus may be delivered using drugs or surgery because it is considered a pursuer trying to kill the mother. However, once its

head has emerged, it may not be harmed because we do not sacrifice one life for another..."

The latitude employed by *halacha* in sanctioning abortion results from this disagreement between Maimonides and Rashi. According to Maimonides, abortion is only allowed as an act of self-defense when the mother's life is at risk, since this is the only circumstance when the fetus can be considered a *rodef.* However, based on Rashi's interpretation, abortion could also be permissible in less dire physical or psychological circumstances that are not necessarily life threatening, since in his view the unborn fetus is not considered a human being on par with the mother. Nevertheless, in both interpretations, it is the mother's status which is the determinant. Based upon Rashi's interpretation, abortion following rape, adultery or other unusual situations could be permitted on a case-by-case basis if the pregnancy were found to cause extreme psychological stress in the mother, whereas abortions for disabled or defective fetuses would generally be forbidden because Judaism considers all life to be of infinite value.

All Orthodox authorities permit, even mandate, abortion in cases of clear danger to the mother's health. In other situations, opinions vary considerably. Former Israeli Chief Rabbi I. Unterman considered abortion "akin to murder" and forbade it under all but the most serious maternal circumstances. R. Feinstein forbade aborting a Tay-Sachs fetus (IM, *Choshen Mishpat* II #69, 70); R. Auerbach also prohibited it but permitted the abortion of an anencephalic fetus (NA, *Choshen Mishpat* 425:1:15; *Orach Chayim* 330:5). Rabbis Waldenberg (TE, IX #51, XIII #102) and Jakobovits, among others, permit abortion in cases of rape or adultery, where the fetus may be severely defective --such as having Tay-Sachs disease or Down's Syndrome -- or if it poses other non-life threatening risks to the mother's physical or mental health. Finally, former Chief Rabbi B.Z. Uziel advocated a more lenient position, permitting abortion in cases where there was a "slim reason" (*ta'am kalush*), such as the prevention of the mother's emotional anguish, shame or disgrace. This view is consistent with earlier precedents allowing abortion in cases characterized by "great emotional pain" (*tzar gufah kadim*) on the part of the mother.

The opinion of the Conservative rabbinate is clear and concise in these matters (CJLS, 1980-85, "Statement on the Permissibility of Abortion"): "Jewish tradition is sensitive to the sanctity of life and does not permit abortion on demand. However, it sanctions abortion under some circumstances because it does not regard the fetus as an autonomous person.... [A]bortion is justifiable if a continuation of pregnancy might cause the mother severe physical or psychological damage, or if the fetus is judged by competent medical opinion to be severely defective. The fetus is a life in the process of development, and the decision to abort should never be taken lightly...." These sentiments are echoed in several Reform responsa (ARR #171; CARR #16; NARR #155).

Although classically, as noted above, the only factor considered when evaluating the permissibility of abortion was the health of the mother, opinions exist in which other determinants were used. Rabbi Isaac Klein, in his *Teshuvah on Abortion*, referred to an earlier responsum that permits abortion in the case of a nursing mother, where the continuation of the pregnancy would have endangered the nursing infant's health. Rabbi Waldenberg has also authorized abortion in cases where "there is substantial risk that the fetus would be born with a deformity that would cause it to suffer" (TE, IX #237).

Other halachic considerations in the prohibition against abortion include the unnecessary destruction of a sperm and egg, intentionally endangering one's life and wounding someone for purposes other than healing. Each of these issues must be factored into individual cases, but they are usually subservient to the overriding concerns of *pikuach nefesh* and the health of the mother.

The fate of the aborted fetus and fetal tissues is also a concern. Although the fetus does not have the status of a person, it does require respectful treatment. R. Caro (Sh Ar,*Yorah Deah* 266) did not require that a fetus be formally buried; yet, R. Feinstein (IM, Yoreh Deah I, #231) insists on the burial of all organs and tissues. In a related issue, since the fetus is not considered a human being, it may be used for experimental research without violating the prohibition of *assur b'hana'ah* (benefiting from the dead) (TE, X #25; CARR #21, and perhaps CJLS 090777, 122788).

The Jewish approach to abortion can perhaps be best summarized as a tension between the right to life, which is absolute, and the right to be born, which is relative (R. I. Klein). All Jewish sources acknowledge the child's right to life at the point at which it is born, after the "majority of the head has emerged from the womb." Judaism does, however, value the life of a human being over other forms of existence such as animal life, plant life or even pre-natal life. Thus, although abortions are permitted by *halacha* under a variety of circumstances, the predominant factors considered relevant by Jewish law relate to the physical or emotional health of the mother, whose status takes precedence over that of the fetus. The status of the fetus and the opinions of the father play lesser roles in this decision. When an abortion is permitted, it should be performed earlier in the pregnancy, preferably within the first 40 days. The halachic approach to abortion confirms the value that Judaism places on actual life over potential life.

## Chapter 7: END OF LIFE ISSUES

*Devorah reluctantly undergoes a therapeutic abortion, but her condition continues to worsen. She understands that there is a reasonable chance that she may die from the complications of her illness. Suddenly she summons all of the emotional strength she has left and expresses interest in preparing an advanced directive.*

No issue in the field of health care affects as many people as the confrontation with death. Whether coping with the untimely demise of a relative or friend, or struggling with the realization of one's own mortality, all of us will eventually find ourselves face to face with death.

Despite this inevitability, few people actually think about, discuss or plan for death in advance, including many that are afflicted with chronic, disabling diseases. In the past, medical science had little to offer critically ill, injured or terminally ill patients, rendering such decisions less important. As technological advances in health care delivery have been made, however, the fate of patients at the end of life has assumed increasing significance. The central role attributed to personal autonomy has led to the development of a means by which patients can declare their personal goals and desires during the final stages of their lives, especially the avoidance of prolonged pain and suffering. The Patient Self-Determination Act of 1991 made this possibility real by requiring that all medical institutions receiving federal funds inform their patients of their right to create an advance directive.

**Issue** Advance directives

**Advance Directives**

Advance directives provide a legal means by which patients can declare their desires for future treatment and care in the event that they become incompetent to make those decisions for themselves. Advance directives take two forms, a living will or a durable power of attorney for health care. A living will is a document in which the patient specifies his or her specific wishes regarding those treatments that they wish to undergo or forego in the event that they are incapacitated. Any and all types of measures can be included, depending upon the patient's preferences. Typical examples include cardiopulmonary resuscitation (CPR), intubation and mechanical ventilation, hemodialysis, artificial feeding, organ donation and autopsy. In contrast, a durable power of attorney for health care, or health care proxy, identifies an individual appointed by the patient to make health care decisions in his or her behalf should they become incompetent. The key charge of the health care proxy, or attorney in fact, is to make health care decisions in accordance with the previously expressed desires of the patient. Thus, it is essential that any person assuming the responsibility of a health care proxy be familiar with the wishes of the patient regarding various options at the end stages of life. Both of these documents are usually invoked by the physician of record, who certifies that the patient is either in a terminal condition (usually defined by statute) or mentally incompetent to make decisions on his own behalf. Also, the patient may revoke an advance directive at any time.

There are advantages and disadvantages to each form of advance directive. Living wills specify in writing the desires of the patient, avoiding confusion. However, it is difficult to anticipate every situation and a living will leaves no room for maneuverability. A durable power of attorney for health care is dynamic, because that decision rests with a person; however, it hinges on that individual's trustworthiness to act in accordance with the patient's wishes and his ability to comprehend the complexities of the situation at hand.

Judaism has a long-standing tradition of individuals expressing their desires before death. In the Torah, this often took the form of blessings, or ethical wills, expressed by the patriarchs to their children. Other famous personalities have bequeathed ethical wills to their children; among the best known was Maimonides. Thus, it is well within Jewish tradition to anticipate death and prepare for it.

In response to the federal mandate, each branch of Judaism has formulated prototype advance directives. Orthodox organizations such as the Rabbinical Council of America and Agudath Israel have each devised advance directives, as have the CJLS (following Rabbis Dorff, Mackler and Reisner) and the Reform movement. The models essentially require that end-of-life decisions be made in accordance with the respective denomination's interpretation of Jewish law and tradition and usually encourage or specify that a rabbi be involved in decision-making.

Physicians are sometimes faced with having to carry out the wishes of a patient specified in an advance directive that are contrary to their own moral or religious beliefs. Most jurisdictions allow physicians that are opposed to the desires of a patient or their health care proxy or the provisions of a living will to transfer the patient to the care of another physician who is sympathetic. In terms of *halacha* and the obligations of Jewish physicians under these circumstances, the answers are unclear. A Jewish doctor is required to act in accordance with Jewish law and respect the sanctity of life at all times. Therefore, would he or she be permitted to transfer a patient to the care of another physician knowing that he or she would act contrary to *halacha*? Does such an act violate the Biblical prohibitions (*Deuteronomy* 19:16) of "*lo ta'amod al dam rei'echa*" ("Do not stand idly by the blood of your neighbor") and "*lifnei iver*" ("Do not place a stumbling block before the blind") (*Leviticus* 19:14)? Rabbis Feinstein and Waldenberg opined that although in theory a physician may treat a patient without his or her consent based upon the above injunction of "*lo ta'amod,*" one is not required to risk his or her life (imprisonment) or livelihood to fulfill that obligation (Rama, Sh Ar, *Yoreh Deah* 336.3; Vilna Gaon commenting on Rama).

The utilization of advance directives in accordance with Jewish law at the end of life reflects the total integration of *halacha* into all aspects of a Jew's life, even those associated with a decision as personal as death.

*Devorah develops severe pneumonia with acute respiratory failure, requiring her to be placed on a mechanical ventilator. Her renal function worsens to the point that her kidney transplant fails and she again needs hemodialysis. She is experiencing considerable discomfort and asks her family if she can be "put out of her misery." By the time they mention this to her doctors, she is unconscious. Her condition is grave and her doctors are beginning to lose hope. They inform the family about Devorah's grim outlook and initiate a discussion about establishing limits for treatment. Gabriel and Devorah's parents begin to feel that as her condition deteriorates her doctors are less available to them. They are angry, hurt and feel abandoned by the professionals they have come to count on over the years.*

Many ethicists and social pundits have commented about the lack of parity between the technical abilities of modern medicine and the ethical principles that govern or modulate their application. Medical science has provided society with enormous opportunities to sustain and prolong life. Many are concerned, though, about the "quality" of such lives, which are, at times, seemingly maintained without regard to the pain and suffering endured by the patients or their families, who are struggling to determine when it is appropriate to withdraw or withhold therapy.

Recently, in Western society, the discussion about withdrawing and withholding medical treatment at the end of life has been expanded to include a debate over euthanasia (derived from the Greek: *eu*- pleasant and *thanatos* - death). Although it is a general term usually understood to mean pleasant or gentle death, several types of euthanasia have been discussed. Active euthanasia, sometimes referred to as "mercy killing," refers to the performance of actions that directly and intentionally result in the death of the individual, such as the administration of a lethal injection. Active-passive euthanasia consists of an action that does not directly cause the death of the patient, such as the removal of life support measures, but results in a situation in which nature takes its course. Passive-passive euthanasia involves a decision to withhold therapy, thereby also allowing the natural history of the disease process to unfold. Physician-assisted suicide is classified as active euthanasia if administered by the physician, or as a suicide if performed by the patient with the physician's involvement limited to writing a prescription for the lethal medication.

**Issues:** Euthanasia, physician-assisted suicide and withdrawing and withholding treatment in the face of pain and suffering

## Euthanasia, Physician-Assisted Suicide and Withdrawing and Withholding Treatment in the Face of Pain and Suffering

"Quality of life," a term commonly used in ethical discussions about matters of life and death, is also important within the Jewish tradition. However, as with most values, Judaism does not regard it as absolute. Instead, "quality of life" must be understood within the context of Judaism's commitment to the "sanctity of life."

The value that Judaism ascribes to human life is exemplified by the Talmudic statement (BT, *Sanhedrin* 37a): "... if anyone caused a single soul to perish, Scripture regards him as if he had caused an entire world to perish; and if anyone saves a single life, Scripture regards him as though he had saved an entire world." Therefore, all Biblical prohibitions, except murder, idolatry and prohibited sexual relations, are suspended in order to save a human life (BT, *Yoma* 82a). However, even the "sanctity of life" is considered a relative value, since the three cardinal offenses in

Judaism that run so counter to that of a moral society may not be committed in order to save one's own life. In such cases, the law is *yaharog v'lo ya'avor,* one is obligated to "be killed rather than transgress." Thus, decisions affecting life and death and the quality of life, or perhaps more aptly, the "quality of death" that one experiences, depend upon balancing a series of relative values.

Judaism distinguishes between the shortening of life (which is forbidden as murder by most authorities) and the prolonging of death (which is also prohibited by most authorities). It is through the interpretation and application of the principle of not prolonging the process of dying that current "quality of life" issues, such as the withholding and withdrawal of treatment -- particularly in the face of intense pain and suffering -- are dealt with.

Every moment of life is considered to be of infinite value in Judaism. Thus, shortening life or hastening death is prohibited. The Bible contains one example of euthanasia, involving the death of King Saul (*Samuel II* 1:1-16). In this account, "the young man [soldier] who brought David the news said: 'I was at Mount Gilboa and saw Saul leaning on his spear as the chariots and horses were closing in on him. He...saw me...and said to me, 'finish me off for I am in agony and barely alive.' '"So I stood over him and finished him off for I knew he would never rise from where he was lying."' After the soldier relates this story to David, he is condemned morally and punished for murder. The conclusion of this episode clearly indicates that active euthanasia is not tolerated in Judaism.

In this regard, the Mishnah (*Semachot* 1:1) states:

> "One who is in a dying condition (*goses* in Hebrew) is considered as a living person in all respects.... One is not permitted to bind his jaws, to stop up his openings, nor place metallic or cooling vessels upon his navel until such time that he dies.... One may not move him, not place him on sand or salt until he dies. One may not close the eyes of a dying person. He who touches them or moves them is shedding blood because R. Meir used to say: 'This can be compared to a flickering flame. As soon as one touches it, it becomes extinguished.' So, whoever closes the eyes of a dying person is regarded as having taken his soul..."

This is reiterated elsewhere in the Talmud (BT, *Shabbat* 151b): "He who closes the eyes of a dying person while the soul is departing is like a murderer. This may be compared to a lamp that is going out. If a man places his finger upon it, it is immediately extinguished."

Maimonides codifies and elaborates on this concept (MT, *Hilchot Avel* 4:5):

> "One who is in a dying condition is regarded as a living person in all respects. It is not permitted to bind his jaws, to stop up the organs of the lower extremities, or to place metallic or cooling vessels upon his navel in order to prevent swelling. He is not to be rubbed or washed, nor is sand or salt to be put upon him until he expires. He who touches him is like one who sheds blood. To what may he be compared? To a flickering flame, which is extinguished as soon as one touches it...."

This is affirmed in the Shulchan Aruch ( *Yoreh Deah* 339).

Furthermore, as noted earlier, the value of human life takes precedence over the laws of the Sabbath (*Pikuach nefesh doche Shabbat*). The Talmud (BT, *Yoma* 85a) states:

> Mishnah: "...every danger to human life suspends [the laws of the] Sabbath. If debris [from a collapsed building] falls on someone and it is doubtful whether he is alive or dead, or whether an Israelite or a heathen, one must probe the heap of the debris for his sake [even on the Sabbath]. If one finds him alive, one should remove the debris but if he is dead, one leaves him there [until after the Sabbath]."

The later codes of Jewish law (MT, *Hilchot Shabbat* 2:1; Sh Ar, *Orach Chayim* 328:4; MB, 328:14) confirm this view.

Yet, the prohibition against shortening life must be balanced against a similar prohibition against prolonging death. The Talmud contains several discussions, both halachic and aggadic, that deal with the subject of death and dying. In discussing the execution of a condemned criminal, the Talmud (BT, *Sanhedrin* 45a, 52a; *Pesachim* 75a) displays sensitivity to the pain associated with the process of dying by requiring that a condemned person be given a potion to dull his or her sensation in order that he have a *mitah yafah* (nice death), in accordance with the commandment "Love your neighbor as yourself" (*Leviticus* 19:25). Rashi interprets *mitah yafah* as meaning a rapid death, implying that the victim not experience prolonged suffering.

The Talmud (BT, *Ketubot* 104a) relates the story of the death of R. Judah HaNasi (the compiler of the Mishnah), who was suffering from a chronic intestinal disorder. The rebbe's disciples continuously prayed for his recovery. His caregiver, witnessing his agony each time he would have to go to the bathroom, remove his phylacteries (*t'fillin*) and replace them, prayed for his death as a relief: "May it be the will of God that the immortals [angels] overpower the mortals [Rebbe's students]." Therefore, she ascended the roof and dropped a large urn. When it shattered, the disciples were distracted from their prayers and the soul of the rebbe was allowed to peacefully depart to heaven. The Talmud in effect praises the rebbe's maidservant for her act of kindness. From this, R. Nissim Gerondi (Ran), in his commentary on the Talmud, infers that it is permitted to pray for death (from God) under similar circumstances.

The story of the death of R. Chanina ben Teradyon (BT, *Avodah Zarah* 18a, Musaf service for Yom Kippur), who was martyred at the hands of the Romans for violating the ban on teaching and studying Torah, also illustrates this principle. After

R. Chanina was captured and sentenced to death, he was wrapped in a Torah scroll with bundles of branches placed around him and set on fire in the presence of his students. The Romans then placed tufts of wool, which were soaked in water over his body so that his death would be prolonged. As he was burning, his disciples called out:

"Rabbi, what do you see?"

R. Chanina answered: "The parchments are being burnt but the letters of the Torah are soaring high."

The students pleaded with him: "Open your mouth so that the fire may enter you [and end your agony]."

R. Chanina replied: "Let He who gave me my soul take it away, but no one should injure oneself."

The Roman executioner, witnessing the conversation, then said to him: "Rabbi, if I raise the flame and remove the tufts of wool from over your heart, will you cause me to enter into the world to come?"

"Yes," the Rabbi replied, after which the executioner hurled himself into the flames with R. Chanina.

Several lessons can be derived from this story. First, great concern was voiced by the students about the severe pain being experienced by R. Chanina. Second, the removal of an impediment to death (the tufts of wool) is permitted in order to allow nature to take its course. However, it is forbidden to hasten one's own death, as R. Chanina refused to open his mouth and allow the flames to enter. Finally, the executioner is ultimately rewarded with entrance into the world to come.

In another anecdote, the Talmud (BT, *Yebamot* 40a) describes an incident in the academy of Rabbi Akiva in which one of his students became seriously ill and none of the others students visited him. When R. Akiva returned from seeing him, he asked the students why they did not fulfill the *mitzvah* of *bikur cholim* (visiting the sick). They answered that there was nothing that they could do. R. Akiva then rebuked his students as follows (according to the Ran): "You could have gone and been of help to him. You could have prayed for his recovery. If you found him in a state of great pain and there was no hope for his recovery, you could have prayed for his speedy death. Even that little help you withheld from him." The issue of psychological trauma is exemplified by the Talmudic legend of Choni the Circle-Drawer (BT, *Ta'anit* 23a), who slept for 70 years. When he awoke and identified himself, no one recognized him or believed him, despite his great mastery of Torah. Because of the extreme mental anguish he suffered, Choni prayed to God for death, and his wish was granted. In a similar story, the *Midrash* describes an old woman that came to R. Yose ben Charlafta saying that she was too old, her life had become meaningless, and she wanted to die. R. Yose asked her how it was that she had lived to such an old age. The woman replied that she attended synagogue services each morning without fail. He then told her to miss three consecutive days. She complied, and died on the third day. These two vignettes highlight the meaning of mental health and the fact that under extreme circumstances, one is permitted to pray for death for the purpose of alleviating emotional anguish.

Based upon these Talmudic sources and a text in the 12th-century work *Sefer Chassidim*, R. M. Isserles, the Rama, prohibited prolongation of the dying process. In his gloss to the *Shulchan Aruch* ( *Orach Chayim* 339:1), he wrote:

> "If there is anything which causes a hindrance to the departure of the soul such as the presence of a knocking noise such as wood chopping near the patient's house or if there is salt on the patient's tongue [in an attempt to revive

him], and these hinder the soul's departure, then it is permissible to remove them because there is no act involved in this at all, but only the removal of the impediment."

The key elements involved in the Rama's ruling, then, are the accurate determination of the point in time when the person's illness has progressed to where death is imminent and our actions are only delaying the "departure of the soul" as well as the nature of the obstacles in question. For example, it seems clear that the sound of wood chopping outside has no therapeutic value, so stopping it should be of no consequence. But, what of removing the salt from the patient's tongue? Is that to be interpreted as withdrawing a medical treatment that is being administered in an attempt to prolong life or is it simply removing an object that serves no therapeutic purpose?

Precise estimation of a prognosis is often not possible, especially in lieu of the current technological advances that are available to prolong the lives of critically and terminally ill patients. The traditional criteria for such a premorbid state (*gesisah*) are that the person is unable to swallow his or her own saliva and that death is imminent within 72 hours. Such a moribund person, known as a *goses,* is considered to be alive in all respects according to *halacha;* no actions may be taken to deliberately hasten death, nor needlessly prolong his life (Mishnah, *Semachot* 1:1, BT; *Shabbat* 151b; MT, *Hilchot Avel* 4:5; Sh Ar, *Yoreh Deah* 339). Several rabbinic authorities have acknowledged, though, that the definition and identification of a *goses* is extremely difficult given modern medical techniques (Rabbis Auerbach, Jakobovits, Dorff). Nevertheless, the concept of being able to withdraw a hindrance to death advanced by the Rama sets an important precedent in resolving these dilemmas according to *halacha*.

Judaism distinguishes between an act of omission (*shev v'al ta'aseh*) and an act of commission (*kum v'aseh*). This is in contrast to general ethics and civil law, in which such a differentiation is irrelevant. Based upon the above Talmudic and halachic sources, it is clear that it is forbidden by Jewish law to commit (*kum v'aseh*) any act that directly shortens the life or hastens the death of any person. However, it is also prohibited to perform any action that prolongs the dying process and increases the pain and suffering of the patient. Thus, the critical issue in each case is whether one can decide if a patient is living or in the act of dying. If the patient is "living," then one must proceed with all available treatments. If the patient is in the act of dying, then one is prohibited from performing any acts that may prolong the process.

Recently, the novel idea that a terminally ill patient is more appropriately categorized as a *t'reifah*, rather than a *goses*, has been proposed (R. Dorff). A *t'reifah* is defined as a person with a known incurable and terminal organic disease who will die within one year, despite human intervention (MT, *Hilchot Rotzeach* 2:8). Such a scenario is quite common in contemporary medicine. The significance of this approach is that the killing of a *t'reifah* is not classified as murder since the *t'reifah* is considered "already dead," whereas a *goses* is considered "alive in all respects."

Many contemporary authorities have issued rulings in this area. R. Feinstein (IM, *Choshen Mishpat* II #73) wrote:

> "Therefore, if a patient is terminally ill and in intractable pain, so that there is no hope of his surviving in a condition free of pain, but it is possible through medical or technological methods to prolong his life, then it is improper to do so. Rather, the patient should be made as comfortable as possible, and left without any further

> intervention.... it is absolutely forbidden to do anything.... that will shorten the patient's life for even a moment."

In such a hopeless situation, R. Feinstein advocates withholding further treatment (*shev v'al ta'aseh*) while strongly reiterating the ban against any act of commission (*kum v'aseh*). Anticipating the ethical "slippery slope" that might derive from his ruling, R. Feinstein (IM, *Choshen Mishpat* II #74) further stated:

> "....in terminal patients, a life of pain need not be preserved. The medical community [you said] will extend this concept to the physically or mentally challenged, and that may lead to involuntary euthanasia.... Nothing in my analysis even hinted at a concept of quality of life which would exclude those who have mental or physical disabilities. It is, or should be, absolutely clear, without any doubt, to anyone who has studied our Torah and who fears Hashem [God], that one must heal or save every individual without any differentiation based upon his intelligence or physical stamina."

This ruling affirms Judaism's commitment to the sanctity of life and *halacha's* categorical opposition to active euthanasia.

R. Chaim David HaLevy, former Chief Rabbi of Tel Aviv, was more lenient in this regard:

> "...permission to remove salt from the tongue is clear....A respirator is exactly the same...The patient was attached [to the respirator] and revived with artificial life in order to try to save him. When the physicians conclude that his condition is hopeless, it is clearly permitted to disconnect him... Indeed, ....if the physicians would wish to persist in keeping him alive on the respirator, it is forbidden to do so... there is a duty not to do so ... since the person's soul, which is God's property, has already been withdrawn."

In his analysis, R. HaLevy relies on the ruling of the Rama that one is forbidden to prolong the dying process, by ordering the removal of the respirator, which HaLevy considers an impediment to death. Disconnecting the respirator allows nature to take its course by creating a situation in which treatment will be omitted (*shev v'al ta'aseh*). However, both R. Feinstein (IM, *Choshen Mishpat* III #132) and R. Waldenberg (TE, XIII #89) only permit discontinuation of mechanical ventilation after it has been established that a patient is halachically dead.

Rabbi Auerbach also ruled that there is no obligation to continue treatment of a suffering terminally ill patient (*Minchat Shlomo* #91:24) and that it is permissible to withdraw certain treatments, such as cardiotonic drugs and hyperalimentation, if they do not precipitate death (NA, *Yoreh Deah* 339:2). However, it should be noted that there are Orthodox authorities that disagree with these interpretations of the Rama's ruling. Rabbis Waldenberg and Bleich are stricter in this regard and believe that aggressive treatment of all terminally ill patients is mandated by *halacha* except for those falling into the category of *goses.*

Conservative and Reform responsa have also sanctioned the withholding or discontinuation of medical treatment in terminally ill patients. Rabbis Dorff and A.I. Reisner, although analyzing terminal illness differently -- with R. Dorff considering the terminally ill patient a *t'reifah* and Reisner considering that person a *goses* -- reached similar conclusions. Artificial interventions, such as mechanical ventilation or hemodialysis, may be withdrawn. Similarly, in several responsa, the Reform rabbinate has concluded that medical treatment may be withheld and withdrawn from terminally ill patients (ARR #77, 78, 79; CARR #83; NARR #156, 159, 160; CCAR 5750.5; 5754.14).

Controversy exists over whether these distinctions apply to a person in a "persistent vegetative state," a permanent, irreversible neurological condition in which a person is able to breathe on his own, but is totally unaware of his surroundings. Such a person cannot communicate or move in any way, eat or even make eye contact. Such patients are comatose yet not "brain dead" and thus cannot serve as organ donors. Strictly speaking, patients in a persistent vegetative state are not considered terminally ill, as they can survive for many years (Karen Ann Quinlan is one example). They also do not suffer from physical or psychological pain. Certainly, they are not in the category of a *goses,* although they could likely be categorized as a *t'reifah.* All Orthodox authorities along with Conservative Rabbi Reisner and members of the Reform rabbinate (CCAR 5750.5) have ruled that all measures must be provided to sustain the life of a patient in a persistent vegetative state. However, R. Dorff of the Conservative movement and Reform Rabbis L. Kravitz, P. Knobel, and Jacob have recently advanced the view that discontinuing care for such patients may be permissible.

Distinct from the question of withholding and withdrawing treatment is the issue of patient autonomy in this area. *Halacha*, by valuing life, views the achievement of long-term survival favorably, making it incumbent on an individual to undergo medical treatment when there is a reasonable chance of achieving *chaye olam* (long life). *Chaye olam* is defined as the patient's having at least a 50 percent chance of surviving one year with functional health, and not in persistent pain and suffering. When such a goal is unattainable, the patient's prognosis is relegated to the category of *chaye sha'ah*, momentary life, and *halacha* recognizes his or her prerogative to exercise considerable autonomy over their treatment. Authorities representing each branch of Judaism have affirmed the patient's prerogative to accept or refuse treatment under these circumstances [Rabbis Feinstein (IM, *Choshen Mishpat* II #73-75); Auerbach (Responsa Yachel Yisrael II #62); Dorff and Reisner (Conservative Judaism 1991); ARR #77, 78, 79; CARR #83, 85; NARR #156, 157, 159, 160; CCAR 5754.14].

A related area in the treatment of the terminally ill deals with the provisions of nutrition and hydration, which is controversial within the general as well as the Jewish community. Because food and water are considered by many to be such basic elements of life, it is viewed as immoral to withhold them from any patient under any circumstances. Most halachic authorities advocate such provisions, with the exception of the case of a *goses* or where the patient specifically refuses [Rabbis Feinstein (IM, *Choshen Mishpat* II #75); Auerbach (Responsa Minchat Shlomo #91:24); Dorff and Reisner (Conservative Judaism 1991); Dorff, *Matters of Life and Death*, pp.208-13; ARR #77; NARR #159; CCAR 5754.14].

Thus, it is apparent that within each branch of Judaism, support exists to varying degrees for both the withdrawal and withholding of treatment from the terminally ill patient who is suffering. Most rabbinic authorities understand these as an example of a *shev v'al ta'aseh* (an act of omission), in which nature is allowed to take its course, and not as a *kum v'aseh*, a deliberate act of commission, which would be classified as active euthanasia or murder. Another interesting framework within which to examine the treatment of the terminally ill is based upon the nature of the practice of medicine (F. Rosner; CCAR 5754.14). In Jewish tradition, the authorization to practice medicine is based upon the presumption that a person will be healed ["heal you shall heal" (*Exodus* 21:19)]. The elevation of the permission to practice medicine to that of an obligation (*mitzvah*), according to Maimonides and Nachmanides, is subsumed by the larger religious duty of *pikuach nefesh* (saving a life). However, as Maimonides codifies the obligation to save a life [(MT, *Hilchot Rotzeach* 1:14), "Whoever is able to save another and does not ......."], the operative word is *able.* That is, the obligation to save the life is dependent upon a reasonable chance of achieving success. If and when that possibility is lost, as in the case of a terminally ill patient, then the obligation to heal, and presumably to accept treatment as well, is also gone. Thus, while there may still be permission to render and accept treatment under these conditions, there would be no obligation (*mitzvah*) to do so. This analysis is consistent with the views of Rabbis Feinstein and HaLevy expressed above.

The prohibition against active euthanasia, which includes physician-assisted suicide, within *halacha* and Jewish tradition has been reaffirmed by authorities from each denomination [Rabbis Feinstein, IM, *Choshen Mishpat* II #73,74; Waldenberg TE V, # 28:5, 29; X #25:6; Dorff and Reisner (Conservative Judaism 1991); ARR #78, 79; CARR #83; NARR #156, 160; CCAR 5750.5; 5754.14]. Thus, the traditional Jewish views concerning euthanasia and the treatment of the terminally ill recognize that motive is important in ethics and may be summarized as follows: Although the outcome is similar, to kill is always wrong, whereas to let someone die is sometimes right and sometimes wrong.

However, there are a number of opinions that support the idea of active euthanasia. In 1952, D.M. Shohet, a Conservative Rabbi, and most recently Rabbis L. Kravitz, P. Knobel, and W. Jacob of the Reform movement have advocated a role for active euthanasia under very specific circumstances and with rigid controls. These arguments are based in part upon the understanding that withdrawal of treatment is, in fact, an active rather than a passive event. Therefore, it is merely semantics, a distinction without a difference, to suggest that turning off a ventilator or discontinuing the administration of drugs, which clearly requires a conscious decision and physical action to bring about, and will result in the death of the individual, are examples of acts of omission (*shev v'al ta'aseh*). In reality, they constitute acts of commission (*kum v'aseh*) and are no different than active euthanasia since the outcome, death, is both known and desired.

Palliative treatment is an important consideration in the management of terminally ill patients, especially those suffering with intense physical pain. In fact, it is the failure to adequately control pain that is most responsible for the current enthusiasm for physician-assisted suicide. Jewish tradition has always taken the mandate to relieve pain seriously, as noted in the Talmudic and Midrashic vignettes described earlier. All rabbinic authorities endorse aggressive treatment of pain in terminally ill patients, even at the risk of inducing respiratory or cardiac depression and precipitating death, provided that the motive is the reduction of pain and not the induction of death (the so-called "double-effect") [Rabbis Feinstein - IM, *Choshen Mishpat* II #73; Waldenberg, TE, XIII # 87; Auerbach, NA,*Yoreh Deah* 339:2; Dorff and Reisner (Conservative Judaism 1991)[9]; ARR #76; CARR #83; NARR #151; CCAR 5754.14]. As a corollary, it is halachically permissible for terminally ill patients to opt for hospice care in order to enhance their pain relief and obtain the necessary emotional support such an environment provides in their final days or weeks of life.

---

9. Rabbi Dorff has written to me stating that he "accepts the 'double effect' argument, Rabbi Avram Reisner does not."

There are some disagreements among well-respected rabbinic decisors in this complex area, reflecting the considerable leeway that exists in the treatment of terminal conditions accompanied by extreme pain and suffering. Such discussions reflect the value that Judaism places on the quality and quantity of life and the value of each individual.

*Devorah's status continues to decline. After extensive deliberations, the decision is made to withhold further aggressive treatment. A week later, Devorah is allowed to die. The doctors are unsure why Devorah's condition deteriorated so rapidly. They are concerned that she may have developed an unusual fatal infection that could affect other transplant patients. In the hope that an examination of Devorah's body could provide important new information that could help them care for other transplant patients, they ask permission to perform an autopsy. Gabriel and Devorah's parents are offended by this request, feeling that it is insensitive and poorly timed.*

An autopsy is a post-mortem examination performed by a pathologist to determine the cause of death. The request for an autopsy may be a relief to a family that is struggling to understand the death of a loved one, or it may be perceived as the height of arrogance and insensitivity by the medical and scientific community, intruding upon the family in its moment of grief.

Post-mortem examinations are responsible for much of what is known today about pathology (the study of disease). Since antiquity, the gross and microscopic study of diseased organs in the patients suffering from numerous infirmities has provided physicians and scientists with critical information. For many years, it was standard for doctors to request an autopsy from the next of kin in all deaths. Over the past few decades, the number of autopsies performed has continually decreased.

**Issues**: Autopsy

**Autopsy**

In general, autopsies are not permitted according to Jewish law because of the principle of *kavod ha'met* (respect for the dead). Respect for the dead has three components: the requirement for rapid burial, prohibition against violating the corpse and the admonition against deriving benefit (*assur b'hana'ah*) from the corpse.

The Torah (*Deuteronomy* 21:22-23) mandates that a dead body be buried quickly: "And if there be a man in sin deserving death, and he be put to death, and you hang him on a tree; his body shall not remain all night upon the tree, but you shall surely bury him that day; for he that is hanged is a reproach to God." Similarly, if an unidentified and unattended dead body is found, the citizens of the nearest town are required to bury it. Even a *Kohen* is permitted to become ritually defiled in order to fulfill this obligation, termed a *met mitzvah* [commandment to bury the dead] (Rashi commenting on *Leviticus* 21:1).

The prohibition against violation of the corpse and deriving *hana'ah* (benefit) from the dead stems from the fact that human beings were created *b'tzelem Elokhim* (in the image of God, *Genesis* 1:27). Therefore, the human body must be treated with respect at all times; failure to do so constitutes a "reproach to God." Just as tattooing, intentionally wounding oneself or creating a bald spot on one's head is forbidden (*Leviticus* 19:27-28; 21:5, *Deuteronomy* 14:1) while one is alive, so too is it prohibited to defile a body that is dead. The body is merely the caretaker of the soul, which belongs to God.

Despite these powerful admonitions against the performance of a post-mortem examination, Jewish tradition recognizes that exceptional circumstances occur. The 18th-century halachist, R. Ezekiel Landau, ruled that an autopsy is permitted in the case of a *choleh le'faneinu* (a sick person immediately before us). That is, if the information will help a sick person who is readily identifiable, then an autopsy is allowed because all laws are suspended in order to save a life (*pikuach nefesh*). However, an autopsy is not permitted if it merely provides medical knowledge that might be valuable in the future. The Conservative movement's CJLS also permits autopsy in cases where the cause of death is unknown, where more than one fatal disease was present or where the final stage of disease brings premature or unexpected death (062060, 111760). The Reform movement, in responsa from 1925 (ARR # 82) and 1986 (CARR #84) concluded that autopsies were permitted in all cases with the consent of the individual while still alive. They felt that a person may forego the honor accorded to a dead person as they would any other honor and that the benefits that would accrue to others justifies such action.

A related issue involves the donation of bodies to medical schools for the study of anatomy. Most Orthodox authorities prohibit the donation or sale of bodies for this purpose (Rabbis Feinstein, Auerbach, Waldenberg, Bleich), citing a violation of *nivul ha'met* (desecration of the corpse) and *ha'na'at ha'met* (deriving benefit from the dead). However, R. Chaim Herzog, the former Chief Rabbi of Israel, permitted it if the deceased freely gave consent while alive and if the organs are carefully preserved for burial. A disagreement among Conservative scholars in this area exists, with the CJLS (112062, 022163, 020666, 010368, 052269) in opposition to the general practice of donation and Rabbis Klein and Dorff adopting a more lenient position. The Reform responsa (ARR #82; CARR #84) do not require burial of all individual organs following an autopsy.

The Jewish views of autopsy and cadaver donation affirm the tradition's respect for the life that was as well as the life that still is.

*Devorah's parents are devastated and brokenhearted by her death. They devoted most of their lives to caring for their sick child and, just as they were hoping that she could begin to have some semblance of a normal life, she was taken from them. They are anguished by what they perceived to be the callousness with which Devorah and they were treated near the end of her life. In addition, they have begun questioning whether closer prenatal and follow-up care could have prevented this final series of complications. Finally, they are quite shocked and overwhelmed at the magnitude of the medical bills for her care, especially since she died despite treatment. For all of these reasons, they are contemplating a medical malpractice lawsuit.*

From the physician's perspective, a claim of malpractice or negligence or a refusal to pay for the medical services rendered when a patient dies may be perceived as the height of arrogance on the part of survivors. Such allegations against physicians take their toll emotionally and professionally. Just as patients and families personalize their medical treatment and outcome, so too do physicians personalize the quality of the health care they provide.

**Issues:** Medical malpractice
Physician fees

## Medical Malpractice and Physician Fees

Obligations entail responsibilities, a statement no less true for physicians than other individuals. It has been recognized in Jewish tradition that doctors have a duty to be as effective as they are able and to provide the highest quality of care possible. A physician is forbidden to administer treatment unless well-versed in both the theory and practice of medicine, and then only when a more competent physician is unavailable. A doctor who practices medicine without a license is liable for any damages resulting from treatment, even if well-acquainted with the field. But, if a physician were mistakenly to cause harm to a patient after having obtained such a license, he would not be held accountable in human courts, though he may still be liable in the heavenly court (Sh Ar *Orach Chayim* 336.1). This "exemption" is granted to physicians because they are necessary *mipnei tikkun haolam* (for the public good) (Tosefta, *Gittin* 4:6). If they were to be held liable for every error, potential doctors would be deterred from entering the profession in the first place.

However, the *Shulchan Aruch* continues, if a licensed practitioner inadvertently causes the death of a patient, he should seek to flee to a city of refuge (*Numbers* 35:9-34), as in a case of manslaughter. There is a debate among commentators about why the penalty for an inadvertent manslaughter is not simply exoneration, as in other cases that occur during the commission of a *mitzvah*, but instead requires exile. One explanation offered is that since the *mitzvah* physicians receive is for healing, if a patient dies, no *mitzvah* was performed; therefore, no exemption exists. Also, an act of murder, which is a capital offense, requires two components, premeditation (*mayzid*) and malice (*ormah*). Clearly, in the case of an inadvertent death caused by a physician, neither of these two components is likely to be present. As a result, Nachmanides, who was also a physician, stated that fear of punishment should not dissuade doctors from treating patients, because only a physician who intentionally causes harm or death to a patient is accountable in a human court.

This view clearly differs from the current American understanding of medical malpractice as well as various ancient views. In ancient Greek law, there was no physician liability, even for intentional murder, whereas in the Code of Hammurabi if a patient died after bloodletting, the physician's hand was severed.

It has been accepted since antiquity that physicians and others may be compensated for services. This principle is based on the Biblical statement (*Leviticus* 25:55): "...for the people of Israel are My servants." In the Talmud (BT, *Bava Kamma* 116b), this was understood to mean "and not the servants of servants," suggesting that people should not be economically beholden to others. Regarding payment of physicians specifically, the Biblical verse "and cause him to be thoroughly healed" (*Exodus* 21:19) has been interpreted as implying that the offender is liable for payment of medical expenses. In addition, the Talmud (*Bava Kamma* 85a) states: "A physician who heals for nothing is worth nothing," expressing concern that one who is not paid for his or her efforts may be less diligent.

A physician may accept remuneration for time and effort spent caring for a patient, but not for giving advice. The act of healing is comparable to returning lost property -- "And you shall restore it to him" (*Deuteronomy* 22:2), an action for which one does not charge a fee. Similarly, Nachmanides (*Torat HaAdam*) applies the Talmudic adage (BT, *Chagigah* 7a), "Just as I, the Lord, act graciously, so should you perform [*mitzvot*] without compensation," to the practice of medicine, suggesting that since the Torah was given to us gratis, so too must we give instruction and advice for free. For this reason, payment for time and effort has always been permitted in an attempt not to deter people from becoming doctors and allowing them to earn a living (Sh Ar, *Yoreh Deah* 336:2; Rama, Sh Ar, *Yoreh Deah* 336:2). In medieval times communities often salaried physicians, paying them from a general fund, to ensure that medical care was always available.

The fee charged should not be excessive and should correspond to what is usual and customary (Sh Ar,*Yoreh Deah* 336:1). However, even if the amount charged by the physician is excessive, the patient is obligated to pay, because the physician sold his or her knowledge, which is beyond ordinary monetary evaluation. Even though healing is a *mitzvah*, the physician is entitled to keep the remuneration because he is not exclusively obligated; the *mitzvah* falls equally to everyone and the physician's payment is therefore not considered illegal usury. Nevertheless, in ancient as well as contemporary times, the status of physicians in the community was controversial. Although frequently praised and held in high esteem, as exemplified by the fact that many of the great Sages of the Talmud and later years

(Maimonides, Nachmanides) were also physicians, this opinion was not universal. The Mishnah (*Kiddushin* 4:14) states: "The best of physicians is destined to Gehenna [hell]". This statement has been interpreted in a variety of ways, but is generally felt to be an admonition against arrogance ("...he who believes he is the best of physicians is destined to Gehenna [hell]") and the notion that it is ultimately the Almighty who heals the sick. Although physicians may be necessary, they must always be cognizant that on their own, they are insufficient to accomplish the sacred task of healing without God's help.

## EPILOGUE

When I began writing this book, I set several goals, which I described to the readers. These aspirations included explaining the workings of Jewish law, allowing people to become more knowledgeable about Judaism, demonstrating that Judaism is a "living entity" capable of meaningfully responding to the most challenging issues of our day, and providing health care professionals with an opportunity to successfully integrate religion into their secular lives and careers without compromising either.

To accomplish my agenda, I utilized a pluralistic approach, including documentation and opinions from each of the branches within contemporary Judaism. During this process, I acquired a tremendous education by uncovering the rich literature that each branch has produced dealing with this subject matter. As a result, I arrived at perhaps the most significant of all realizations – that, despite the seemingly irreconcilable differences and conflicts that exist in contemporary Jewry, both within and between individual branches, a spark of hope exists. Contrary to what one might anticipate at the outset, there exists a remarkable unanimity of opinion among the different branches about many of the ethical dilemmas that have been discussed here. In the end, this is not really surprising because all of the streams within Judaism share a remarkable agreement -- that the ethical commandments in the Torah are eternal and binding.

Studying the commonalities and differences among these approaches has implications for our understanding and dealing with the contemporary Jewish scene. One could conclude, in the most idealistic light, that the Talmudic dictum: "These and these are the words of the living God" (BT, *Eruvin* 13b) applies, suggesting that they are simply different, but equally legitimate, analyses. Such an interpretation, while acceptable to some, would surely be rejected by others.

A more appropriate example might be the famous Talmudic discussion concerning the proper manner in which one describes a bride at her wedding (BT, *Ketubot* 16b, 17a):

"The Rabbis taught: 'How does one dance before a bride?' The House of Shammai states: '[One describes] the bride as she appears.' The House of Hillel answers: [Every bride is a] 'beautiful and graceful bride.'

The House of Shammai said to the House of Hillel: 'If she was lame or blind, does one [still] say of her: 'Beautiful and graceful bride,' as the Torah (*Exodus* 23:7) states, 'Keep far from falsehood'?

Replied the House of Hillel to the House of Shammai: 'According to your reasoning, if one has made a bad purchase in the market, should one praise it in his [the purchaser's] eyes or depreciate it? Surely, one should praise it in his eyes. Therefore, the Sages said: 'The disposition of man should always be pleasant with people… '''

Since the rule is in accordance with the view of the House of Hillel, this anecdote suggests that each denomination should be comfortable and proud of its achievements in the ethical arena and that the others should recognize, appreciate and emphasize the positive contributions inherent in each. So much has been made of the differences within Jewry today that it has become too easy to lose sight of the fact that there is still more that unites us as Jews than divides us.

There is a well-known saying that optimists see the glass as half full, while pessimists see it as half empty. Without underestimating or minimizing the issues that divide contemporary Jewry, it appears to me that each branch has remained true not only to itself – but to Jewish tradition -- in its approach to the complex ethical dilemmas. If nothing else, this approach has shown me that the glass is indeed half full.

# REFERENCES

## Chapter 1: Selected References – Origins And Definition of Jewish Medical Ethics

Barcalow, E. *Moral Philosophy: Theory and Issues*. Belmont, Ca.: Wadsworth Publishing Co., 1994.

Beauchamp, T.L. and Childress, J.F. *Principles of Biomedical Ethics* (2nd ed.), New York: Oxford University Press, 1996.

Bleich, J.D. "The A Priori Component of Bioethics." In *Jewish Bioethics*, edited by F. Rosner and J.D. Bleich. New York: Hebrew Publishing Co.., 1979.

Dorff, E.N. *Matters of Life and Death: A Jewish Approach to Modern Medical Ethics.* Philadelphia: Jewish Publication Society, 1998.

Dorff, E.N. and Newman, L.E. (Eds). *Contemporary Jewish Ethics and Morality: A Reader.* New York: Oxford University Press, 1995.

Glick, S. "Trends in Medical Ethics in a Pluralistic Society: A Jewish Perspective." Seventeenth Annual Rabbi Louis Feinberg Memorial Lecture in Judaic Studies, University of Cincinnati, Cincinnati, Ohio, April 1994.

Jakobovits, I. *Jewish Medical Ethics.* New York: Bloch Publishing, 1974.

Knobel, P. "Suicide, Assisted Suicide, Active Euthanasia: A Halakhic Inquiry." In *Death and Euthanasia in Jewish Law: Essays and Responsa*, edited by W. Jacob and M. Zemer. Pittsburgh: Freehof Institute of Progressive Halachah, 1995.

Sacks, J. *Arguments for the Sake of Heaven: Emerging Trends in Traditional Judaism.* Northvale, N.J.: Jason Aronson, Inc., 1991.

Steinberg, A. "Medical Ethics: Secular and Jewish Approaches." In *Medicine and Jewish Law* (I), edited by F. Rosner. Northvale, N.J.: Jason Aronson, Inc., 1991.

Wurzburger, W.S. *Ethics of Responsibility: Pluralistic Approaches to Covenantal Ethics.* Philadelphia: Jewish Publication Society, 1994.

Zohar, N.J. *Alternatives in Jewish Bioethics.* Albany: State University of New York Press, 1997.

Zoloth-Dorfman, L. "Face to Face, Not Eye to Eye: Further Conversations on Jewish Medical Ethics." *Journal of Clinical Ethics* 6:222-231 (1995).

## Chapter 2: Selected References - Overview of Jewish Law

Bleich, J.D. *Contemporary Halakhic Problems (Vol 1).* New York: Ktav Publishing & Yeshiva University Press, 1977.

Dorff, E.N. *Conservative Judaism: Our Ancestors to Our Descendants.* New York: United Synagogue of America, 1977.

Dorff, E.N. *Matters of Life and Death: A Jewish Approach to Modern Medical Ethics.* Philadelphia: Jewish Publication Society, 1998.

Dorff, E.N. and Newman, L.E. (Eds). *Contemporary Jewish Ethics and Morality: A Reader.* New York: Oxford University Press, 1995.

Elon, M. *The Principles of Jewish Law.* (Encyclopedia Judaica). Jerusalem: Keter Publishing House, 1994.

Feldman, D.M. *Marital Relations, Birth Control and Abortion in Jewish Law.* (3rd ed). New York: New York University Press, 1995.

Jakobovits, I. *Jewish Medical Ethics.* New York: Bloch Publishing, 1974.

Knobel, P. "Suicide, Assisted Suicide, Active Euthanasia: A Halakhic Inquiry." In *Death and Euthanasia in Jewish Law: Essays and Responsa*, edited by W. Jacob and M. Zemer. Pittsburgh: Freehof Institute of Progressive Halachah, 1995.

Landesman, D. *A Practical Guide to Torah Learning*. Northvale, N.J.: Jason Aronson, Inc., 1995.

Rosner, F. *Pioneers in Jewish Medical Ethics*. Northvale, N.J.: Jason Aronson, Inc., 1998.

Telushkin, J. *Jewish Literacy*. New York: William Morrow and Co., 1991.

Washofsky, M. "Abortion and the Halachic Conversation: A Liberal Perspective." In *Fetus and Fertility in Jewish Law: Essays and Responsa*, edited by W. Jacob and M. Zemer. Pittsburgh: Freehof Institute of Progressive Halachah, 1995.

Zohar, N.J. *Alternatives in Jewish Bioethics*. Albany: State University of New York Press, 1997.

## Chapter 3: Selected References: Religious Denominations in Contemporary Judaism

Dorff, E.N. *Conservative Judaism: Our Ancestors to Our Descendants*. New York: United Synagogue of America, 1977.

Knobel, P. "Suicide, Assisted Suicide, Active Euthanasia: A Halakhic Inquiry." In *Death and Euthanasia in Jewish Law: Essays and Responsa*, edited by W. Jacob and M. Zemer. Pittsburgh: Freehof Institute of Progressive Halachah, 1995.

Rosenthal, G.S. *The Many Faces of Judaism: Orthodox, Conservative, Reconstructionist & Reform*. West Orange, N.J.: Behrman House, Inc., 1978.

Sacks, J. *Arguments for the Sake of Heaven: Emerging Trends in Traditional Judaism.* Northvale, N.J.: Jason Aronson, Inc., 1991.

Telushkin, J. *Jewish Literacy*. New York: William Morrow and Co., 1991.

## Chapter 4: ROLES AND RESPONSIBILITIES

### Selected References: Role of God in Illness and Healing


Berkovits, E. *Faith After the Holocaust*. New York: Ktav Publishing, 1973.

Bleich, J.D. *Judaism and Healing: Halachic Perspectives*. New York: Ktav Publishing, 1981.

Bulka, R.P. *Judaism on Illness and Suffering*. Northvale, N.J.: Jason Aronson, Inc., 1998.

Cohen, A.A., and Mendes-Flohr, P. (Eds). *Contemporary Jewish Religious Thought.* New York: Free Press, 1977.

Dorff, E.N. *Matters of Life and Death: A Jewish Approach to Modern Medical Ethics.* Philadelphia: Jewish Publication Society, 1998.

Greenberg, I. *The Jewish Way*. New York: Simon and Shuster, 1988.

Isaacs, R.H. *Judaism, Medicine and Healing.* Northvale, N.J.: Jason Aronson, Inc., 1998.

Jakobovits, I. *Jewish Medical Ethics*. New York: Bloch Publishing, 1974.

Kushner, H.S. *When Bad Things Happen to Good People.* New York: Schocken Press, 1981.

Rosner, F. *Modern Medicine and Jewish Ethics*. New York: Ktav Publishing, 1991.

Rosner, F. and Bleich, J.D. (Eds). *Jewish Bioethics*. New York: Hebrew Publishing Co.., 1979.

Rubenstein, R.L. *After Auschwitz: History, Theology, and Contemporary Judaism* (2nd ed). Baltimore: Johns Hopkins University Press, 1992.

Telushkin, J. *Jewish Literacy*. New York: William Morrow and Co., 1991.

Zohar, N.J. *Alternatives in Jewish Bioethics*. Albany: State University of New York Press, 1997.

**Selected References: Obligation of Patients to Undergo Treatment**

Bleich, J.D. *Judaism and Healing: Halachic Perspectives*. New York: Ktav Publishing, 1981.

Bleich, J.D. "The Obligation to Heal in the Judaic Tradition: A Comparative Analysis." In *Jewish Bioethics*, edited by F. Rosner and J.D. Bleich. New York: Hebrew Publishing Co.., 1979.

Bulka, R.P. *Judaism on Illness and Suffering.* Northvale, N.J.:Jason Aronson, Inc., 1998.

Dorff, E.N. *Matters of Life and Death: A Jewish Approach to Modern Medical Ethics.* Philadelphia: Jewish Publication Society, 1998.

Dorff, E.N. and Newman, L.E. (Eds). *Contemporary Jewish Ethics and Morality: A Reader.* New York: Oxford University Press, 1995.

Isaacs, R.H. *Judaism, Medicine and Healing.* Northvale, N.J.: Jason Aronson, Inc., 1998.

Jakobovits, I. *Jewish Medical Ethics.* New York: Bloch Publishing, 1974.

Koenigsberg, M. *Halachah & Medicine Today.* New York: Feldheim Publishers, 1997.

Rosner, F. "The Physician and the Patient in Jewish Law." In *Jewish Bioethics*, edited by F. Rosner and J.D. Bleich. New York: Hebrew Publishing Co.., 1979.

Rudman, Z.C. "Fetal Rights and Maternal Obligations." *J. Halacha and Contemporary Society* XIII (1987): 113-124.

**Selected References: Role and Responsibility of Physicians in Healing**

Bleich, J.D. *Judaism and Healing: Halachic Perspectives*. New York: Ktav Publishing, 1981.

Bleich, J.D. "The Obligation to Heal in the Judaic Tradition: A Comparative Analysis." In *Jewish Bioethics*, edited by F. Rosner and J.D. Bleich. New York: Hebrew Publishing Co.., 1979.

Bulka, R.P. *Judaism on Illness and Suffering*. Northvale, N.J.: Jason Aronson, Inc., 1998.

Dorff, E.N. *Matters of Life and Death: A Jewish Approach to Modern Medical Ethics*. Philadelphia: Jewish Publication Society, 1998.

Dorff, E.N. and Newman, L.E. (Eds). *Contemporary Jewish Ethics and Morality: A Reader*. New York: Oxford University Press, 1995.

Isaacs, R.H. *Judaism, Medicine and Healing*. Northvale, N.J.: Jason Aronson, Inc., 1998.

Jakobovits, I. *Jewish Medical Ethics*. New York: Bloch Publishing, 1974.

Koenigsberg, M. *Halachah & Medicine Today*. New York: Feldheim Publishers, 1997.

Rosner, F. "Physician's Strikes and Jewish Law." *J. Halacha and Contemporary Society* XXV (1993): 37-48.

Rosner, F. "The Physician and the Patient in Jewish Law." In *Jewish Bioethics,* edited by F. Rosner and J.D. Bleich. New York: Hebrew Publishing Co., 1979.

Rosner, F. (translator). *Julius Preuss' Biblical and Talmudic Medicine*. Northvale, N.J.: Jason Aronson, Inc., 1993.

Rosner, F. *Modern Medicine and Jewish Ethics*. New York: Ktav Publishing, 1991.

Rudman, Z.C. "Fetal Rights and Maternal Obligations." *J. Halacha and Contemporary Society* XIII (1987): 113-124.

**Selected References: Beneficence, Paternity and Autonomy**

Barcalow, E. *Moral Philosophy: Theory and Issues*. Belmont, CA: Wadsworth Publishing Co., 1994.

Beauchamp, T.L. and Childress, J.F. *Principles of Biomedical Ethics* (2nd ed.). New York: Oxford University Press, NY.

Bleich, J.D. *Judaism and Healing: Halachic Perspectives*. New York: Ktav Publishing, 1981.

Bleich, J.D. *Judaism and Healing: Halachic Perspectives*. New York: Ktav Publishing, 1981.

Bleich, J.D. "The Obligation to Heal in the Judaic Tradition: A Comparative Analysis." In *Jewish Bioethics,* edited by F. Rosner and J.D. Bleich. New York: Hebrew Publishing Co., 1979.

Dorff, E.N. *Matters of Life and Death: A Jewish Approach to Modern Medical Ethics.* Philadelphia: Jewish Publication Society, 1998.

Glick, S. "Trends in Medical Ethics in a Pluralistic Society: A Jewish Perspective." Seventeenth Annual Rabbi Louis Feinberg Memorial Lecture in Judaic Studies, University of Cincinnati, Cincinnati, Ohio, April 1994.

Jakobovits, I. *Jewish Medical Ethics*. New York: Bloch Publishing, 1974.

Rosner, F. "The Physician and the Patient in Jewish Law." In *Jewish Bioethics,* edited by F. Rosner and J.D. Bleich. New York: Hebrew Publishing Co., 1979.

Rosner, F. *Modern Medicine and Jewish Ethics*. New York: Ktav Publishing, 1991.

Rosner, F. (Ed.) *Medicine and Jewish Law* (I & II). Northvale, N.J.: Jason Aronson, Inc., 1991, 1993.

Rudman, Z.C. "Fetal Rights and Maternal Obligations." *J. Halacha and Contemporary Society* XIII (1987): 113-124.

Wurzburger, W.S. *Ethics of Responsibility: Pluralistic Approaches to Covenantal Ethics.* Philadelphia: Jewish Publication Society, 1994.

Zohar, N.J. *Alternatives in Jewish Bioethics.* Albany: State University of New York Press, 1997.

**Selected References: The Role of the Rabbi in Medical Decision-Making**

Grodin, M.A. "Halakhic Dilemmas in Modern Medicine." *J. Clinical Ethics* 6 (1995): 218-221.

Keilson, M. "A Physician's Dilemma: Which Rabbinic Decisor to Ask." In *Medicine and Jewish Law* (Vol. II), edited by F. Rosner. Northvale, N.J.: Jason Aronson, Inc., 1993

Wein, B. "Rabbinic Decision-Making in Medical Practice: The Rabbis's Perspective." In *Medicine and Jewish Law* (Vol. II), edited by F. Rosner. Northvale, N.J.: Jason Aronson, Inc., 1993.

## Chapter 5: ISSUES IN THE TREATMENT OF ILLNESS

### Selected References: Sanctity of Life and Violation of the Sabbath to Save a Life

Abraham, A.S. *Comprehensive Guide to Medical Halachah.* New York: Feldheim Publishers, 1990.

Abraham, A.S. "The Patient on the Sabbath." In *Medicine and Jewish Law* (Vol. I), edited by F. Rosner. Northvale, N.J.: Jason Aronson, Inc., 1991.

Abraham, A.S. "The Jewish Physician and the Sabbath." In *Medicine and Jewish Law* (Vol II), edited by F. Rosner. Northvale, N.J.: Jason Aronson, Inc., 1993.

Bleich, J.D. *Judaism and Healing: Halachic Perspectives*. New York: Ktav Publishing, 1981.

Bleich, J.D. *Contemporary Halakhic Problems* (Vol I, IV). New York: Ktav Publishing & Yeshiva University Press, 1977, 1995.

Dorff, E.N. *Matters of Life and Death: A Jewish Approach to Modern Medical Ethics.* Philadelphia: Jewish Publication Society, 1998.

Jakobovits, I. *Jewish Medical Ethics.* New York: Bloch Publishing, 1974.

Koenigsberg, M. *Halachah & Medicine Today.* New York: Feldheim Publishers, 1997.

Rosner, F. "The Jewish Attitude Toward Euthanasia." In *Jewish Bioethics,* edited by F. Rosner and J.D. Bleich. New York: Hebrew Publishing Co., 1979.

Rosner, F. *Modern Medicine and Jewish Ethics.* New York: Ktav Publishing, 1991.

Rosner, F. and Tendler, M.D. *Practical Medical Halachah.* Northvale, N.J.: Jason Aronson, Inc., 1997.

Rosner, F. *Pioneers in Jewish Medical Ethics.* Northvale, N.J.: Jason Aronson, Inc., 1998.

**Selected References: "Experimental" or Newer Treatments**

Abraham, A.S. *Comprehensive Guide to Medical Halachah.* New York: Feldheim Publishers, 1990.

Bleich, J.D. "Experiments on Human Subjects." In *Jewish Bioethics*, edited by F.Rosner and J.D. Bleich. New York: Hebrew Publishing Co.., 1979.

Bleich, J.D. *Judaism and Healing: Halachic Perspectives.* New York: Ktav Publishing, 1981.

Bleich, J.D. *Contemporary Halakhic Problems* (Vol II, III, IV). New York: Ktav Publishing & Yeshiva University Press, 1983, 1989, 1995.

Cohen, D. "Taking Risks." *J. Halacha and Contemporary Society* XXXIII (1997): 37-70.

Dorff, E.N. *Matters of Life and Death: A Jewish Approach to Modern Medical Ethics.* Philadelphia: Jewish Publication Society, 1998.

Jakobovits, I. *Jewish Medical Ethics.* New York: Bloch Publishing, 1974.

Jakobovits, I. "Medical Experiments on Humans in Jewish Law." In *Jewish Bioethics*, edited by F. Rosner and J.D. Bleich. New York: Hebrew Publishing Co., 1979.

Rosner, F. "Judaism and Human Experimentation." In *Jewish Bioethics*, edited by F. Rosner and J.D. Bleich. New York: Hebrew Publishing Co., 1979.

Rosner, F. *Modern Medicine and Jewish Ethics.* New York: Ktav Publishing, 1991.

**Selected References: Genetic Engineering**

Bleich, J.D. *Judaism and Healing: Halachic Perspectives*. New York: Ktav Publishing, 1981.

Dorff, E.N. *Matters of Life and Death: A Jewish Approach to Modern Medical Ethics.* Philadelphia: Jewish Publication Society, 1998.

Rosner, F. *Modern Medicine and Jewish Ethics.* New York: Ktav Publishing, 1991.

**Selected References: Unethical Conduct of Physicians and Scientists During the Holocaust**

Aly, G., Chroust, P., and Pross, C. *Cleansing the Fatherland.* Baltimore: Johns Hopkins University Press, 1994.

Annas, G.L.J., Grodin, M.A. (Eds). *The Nazis and the Nuremberg Code: Human Rights in Human Experimentation.* New York: Oxford University Press, 1992.

Burleigh, M. *Death and Deliverance: Euthanasia in Germany, 1900-1945.* Cambridge, England: Cambridge University Press, 1994.

Caplan, A.L. (Ed). *When Medicine Went Mad: Bioethics and the Holocaust*. Totowa, N.J.: Humana Press, 1992.

Gallagher, H. *By Trust Betrayed: Patients, Physicians and the License to Kill in the Third Reich.* New York: Holt and Co., 1990.

Goldhagen, D.J. *Hitler's Willing Executioners: Ordinary Germans and the Holocaust*. New York: Alfred A. Knopf, 1996.

Hilberg, R. *Perpetrators, Victims, Bystanders: The Jewish Catastrophe 1933-1945.* New York: Harper Collins, 1992.

Kater, M. *Doctors under Hitler*. Chapel Hill: University of North Carolina Press, 1989.

Lifton R.J. *The Nazi Doctors: Medical Killing and the Psychology of Genocide*. New York: Basic Books, 1986.

Michalczyk, J.J. (Ed.). *Medicine, Ethics and the Third Reich: Historical and Contemporary Issues*. Kansas City, Mo.: Sheed and Ward, 1994.

Mitscherlich, A., and Mielke, F. *Doctors of Infamy: The Story of Nazi Medical Crimes*. New York: H. Schumman, 1949.

Muller-Hill, B. *Murderous Science: Elimination by Scientific Selection of Jews, Gypsies and Others in Germany 1933-1945*. Oxford, England: Oxford University Press, 1988.

Nyiszli, M. *Auschwitz: A Doctor's Eyewitness Account*. New York: Arcade Publishing, 1960, 1993 (English).

Proctor, R.N. *Racial Hygiene: Medicine Under the Nazis*. Cambridge, Mass.: Harvard University Press, 1988.

Sereny, G. *Into That Darkness: From Mercy Killing to Mass Murder*. New York: McGraw-Hill, 1974.

Shelley, L. *Criminal Experiments on Human Beings in Auschwitz and War Research Laboratories: Twenty Women Prisoners' Accounts*. San Francisco: Mellon Research University Press, 1991.

**Selected Journal Articles**

Alexander, L.. "Medical Science Under Dictatorship." *NEJM* 241 (1949): 39-47.

Barondess, J.A. "Medicine Against Society: Lessons from the Third Reich." *JAMA* 276 (1996): 1657-1661.

Berger, R. "Nazi Science-The Dachau Hypothermia Experiments." *NEJM* 322 (1990): 1435-1440.

Caplan, A.L.. "The Meaning of the Holocaust for Bioethics." *Hastings Center Report* 19 (1989): 2-3.

Gutman, I. (Ed). "Medical Experiments." *Encyclopedia of the Holocaust,* Vol. 3 (1990): 957-966.

Hanauske-Abel, H.M. "From Holocaust to Nuclear Holocaust: A Lesson to Learn?" *Lancet* (Aug. 2, 1986): 271-273.

Hanauske-Abel, H.M. "Not a Slippery Slope Subversion: German Medicine and National Socialism in 1933." *BMJ* 313 (1996): 1453-1463.

Leasing, J. "War Crimes and Medical Science." *BMJ* 313 (1996): 1413-1415.

Proctor, R.N. "The Anti-tobacco Campaign of the Nazis: a Little Known Aspect of Public Health in Germany, 1933-45." *BMJ* 313 (1996): 1450-1453.

Pross, C. "Breaking Through Postwar Corruption of Nazi Doctors in Germany." *J. Med Ethics* 17 (1991): 13-16.

Seidelman, W.E. "Mengele Medicus: Medicine's Nazi Heritage." *Int. J. Health Svcs.* 19 (1989): 599-610.

Seidelman, W.E. "In Memoriam: Medicine's Confrontation with Evil." *Hastings Center Report* 19 (1989): 5-6.

Seidelman W.E. "The path to Nuremberg in the pages of J.A.M.A. 1933 -1939." *JAMA* 276 (1996): 1693-1696.

Seidelman, W.E. "Nuremberg Lamentation: for the Forgotten Victims of Medical Science." *BMJ* 313 (1996): 1463-1467.

Shevell, M. "Racial Hygiene, Active Euthanasia, and Julius Hallervorden." *Neurology* 42 (1992): 2212-2219.

**Selected References: Proper Conduct of Human Experiments**

Bleich, J.D. "Experiments on Human Subjects." In *Jewish Bioethics*, edited by F. Rosner and J.D. Bleich. New York: Hebrew Publishing Co., 1979.

Faden, R., Lederer, S.E., and Moreno, J.d. "U.S. Medical Researchers, the Nuremberg Doctors Trial, and the Nuremberg Code: Findings of the Advisory Committee on Human Radiation Experiments." *JAMA* 276 (1996): 1667-1671.

Hanauske-Abel, H.M. "Not a Slippery Slope Subversion: German Medicine and National Socialism in 1933." *BMJ* 313 (1996): 1453-1463.

Harkness, J. "Nuremberg and the Issue of Wartime Experiments on U.S. Prisoners: the Green Committee." *JAMA* 276 (1996): 1672-1675.

Katz, J. "The Nuremberg Code and the Nuremberg Trial: A Reappraisal." *JAMA* 276 (1996): 1662-1666.

Sidel, V. "The Social Responsibilities of Health Professionals: Lessons from Their Role in Nazi Germany." *JAMA* 276 (1996): 1679-1681.

Vollmann, J., Winau, R. "Informed Consent in Human Experimentation Before the Nuremberg Code." *BMJ* 313 (1996): 1444-1447.

Weindling, P. "Human Guinea Pigs and the Ethics of Experimentation: the Bmjs Correspondent at the Nuremberg Medical Trial." *BMJ* 313 (1996): 1467-1470.

**Selected References: Use of Improperly Obtained Scientific Data**

Angell, M. "The Nazi Hypothermia Experiments and Unethical Research Today" (Editorial). *NEJM* 322 (1990): 1462-1464.

Bleich, J.D. "Utilization of Scientific Data Obtained Through Immoral Experimentation." *Tradition* 26 (1991): 65-75.

Faden, R., Lederer, S.E., and Moreno, J.D. "U.S. Medical Researchers, the Nuremberg Doctors Trial, and the Nuremberg Code: Findings of the Advisory Committee on Human Radiation Experiments." *JAMA* 276 (1996): 1667-1671.

Moe, K. "Should the Nazi Research Data Be Cited?" *Hastings Center Report* 14 (1984): 5-7.

Post, S.G. "The Echo of Nuremberg: Nazi Data and Ethics." *J. Med Ethics* 17 (1991): 42-44.

Sheldon, M. "Nazi Data: Dissociation from Evil." *Hastings Center Report* 19 (1989): 16-18.

## Selected References: Triage, Rationing and Allocation of Medical Resources

Abraham, A.S. "Priorities in Medicine: Whom to Treat First" in *Medicine and Jewish Law* (I), edited by F. Rosner. Northvale, N.J.: Jason Aronson, Inc., 1991.

Bleich, J.D. "Medical and Life Insurance: A Halachic Mandate." *Tradition* 31 (1997): 52-70.

Dorff, E.N. *Matters of Life and Death: A Jewish Approach to Modern Medical Ethics.* Philadelphia: Jewish Publication Society, 1998.

Jakobovits, I. *Jewish Medical Ethics.* New York: Bloch Publishing, 1974.

**Selected References: Suicide**

Bleich, J.D. *Judaism and Healing: Halachic Perspectives*. New York: Ktav Publishing, 1981.

Dorff, E.N. *Matters of Life and Death: A Jewish Approach to Modern Medical Ethics*. Philadelphia: Jewish Publication Society, 1998.

Dorff, E.N. "Teshuvah on Assisted Suicide." *Conservative Judaism* 50 (1988): 3-24.

Herring, B.F. *Jewish Ethics and Halachah for Our Time*. New York: Yeshiva University Press, 1984.

Jakobovits, I. *Jewish Medical Ethics*. New York: Bloch Publishing, 1974.

Prouser, J.H. "Being of Sound Mind and Judgement: Rethinking Sanctions in the Case of Physician Assisted Suicide." *Conservative Judaism* 49 (1997): 3-16.

Rosner, F. "Suicide in Jewish Law" in *Jewish Bioethics*, edited by F. Rosner and J.D. Bleich. New York: Hebrew Publishing Co.., 1979.

Rosner, F. *Modern Medicine and Jewish Ethics*. New York: Ktav Publishing, 1991.

Siegel, S. "Suicide in the Jewish View." *Conservative Judaism* 32 (1979): 67.

**Selected References: Harmful Behaviors - Smoking**

Bleich, J.D. Smoking. *Tradition* 16 (1977):121-125.

Dorff, E.N. *Matters of Life and Death: A Jewish Approach to Modern Medical Ethics.* Philadelphia: Jewish Publication Society, 1998.

Herring, B.F. *Jewish Ethics and Halachah for Our Time.* New York: Yeshiva University Press, 1984.

Jakobovits, I. *Jewish Medical Ethics.* New York: Bloch Publishing, 1974.

Rosner, F. *Modern Medicine and Jewish Ethics.* New York: Ktav Publishing, 1991.

Slae, M. *Smoking and Damage to Health in the Halachah.* Jerusalem: Acharai Publications, 1990.

**Selected References: Harmful Behaviors – Alcohol and Illicit Drugs**

Bleich, J.D. *Judaism and Healing: Halachic Perspectives.* New York: Ktav Publishing, 1981.

Brayer, M.M. "Drugs: A Jewish View." In *Jewish Bioethics*, edited by F. Rosner and J.D. Bleich. New York: Hebrew Publishing Co., 1979.

Dorff, E.N. *Matters of Life and Death: A Jewish Approach to Modern Medical Ethics.* Philadelphia: Jewish Publication Society, 1998.

Herring, B.F. *Jewish Ethics and Halachah for Our Time.* New York: Yeshiva University Press, 1984.

Jakobovits, I. *Jewish Medical Ethics.* New York: Bloch Publishing, 1974.

Rosner, F. *Modern Medicine and Jewish Ethics.* New York: Ktav Publishing, 1991.

Spero, M.H. *Judaism and Psychology: Halachic Perspectives.* New York: Ktav Publishing, Yeshiva University Press, 1980.

**Selected References: Psychiatric Care**

Bleich, J.D. *Judaism and Healing: Halachic Perspectives.* NewYork: Ktav Publishing, 1981.

Jakobovits, I. *Jewish Medical Ethics.* New York: Bloch Publishing, 1974.

Rosner, F. *Modern Medicine and Jewish Ethics.* New York: Ktav Publishing, 1991.

Smith, N. "Psychiatric Issues Confronting the Practicing Physician." In *Medicine and Jewish Law* (II), edited by F. Rosner. Northvale, N.J.: Jason Aronson, Inc., 1993.

Spero, M.H. "Psychiatry, Psychotherapy and Halachah." In *Jewish Bioethics,* edited by F. Rosner and J.D. Bleich. New York: Hebrew Publishing Co., 1979.

Tendler, M.D. "The Halachic Import of the Psychological State." In *Medicine and Jewish Law* (II), edited by F. Rosner. Northvale, N.J.: Jason Aronson, Inc., 1993.

**Selected References: Permissibility of Organ Transplantation**

Bleich, J.D. *Contemporary Halakhic Problems* (Vol I, III, IV). New York: Ktav Publishing & Yeshiva University Press, 1977, 1989, 1995.

Bleich, J.D. "Establishing Criteria of Death." In *Jewish Bioethics*, edited by F. Rosner and J.D. Bleich. New York: Hebrew Publishing Co., 1979.

Bleich, J.D. "Neurological Death and Time of Death Statutes." In *Jewish Bioethics,* edited by F. Rosner and J.D. Bleich. New York: Hebrew Publishing Co., 1979.

Bleich, J.D. *Judaism and Healing: Halachic Perspectives*. New York: Ktav Publishing, 1981.

Dorff, E.N. *Matters of Life and Death: A Jewish Approach to Modern Medical Ethics.* Philadelphia: Jewish Publication Society, 1998.

Jakobovits, I. *Jewish Medical Ethics*. New York: Bloch Publishing, 1974.

Rabinovitch, N.L. "What is Halachah for Organ Transplants?" in *Jewish Bioethics,* edited by F. Rosner and J.D. Bleich. New York: Hebrew Publishing Co., 1979.

Rosner, F. "Organ Transplantation in Jewish Law" in *Jewish Bioethics*, edited by F. Rosner and J.D. Bleich. New York: Hebrew Publishing Co., 1979.

Rosner, F. *Modern Medicine and Jewish Ethics*. New York: Ktav Publishing, 1991.

Soloveichik, A. "The Halachic Definition of Death." In *Jewish Bioethics*, edited by F. Rosner and J.D. Bleich. New York: Hebrew Publishing Co.., 1979.

Steinberg, A. "The Definition of Death." In *Medicine and Jewish Law* (I), edited by F. Rosner. Northvale, N.J.: Jason Aronson, Inc., 1991.

Tendler, M.D. *Responsa of Rabbi Moshe Feinstein: Critical Illness* (Vol 1). New York: Ktav Publishing, 1996.

**Selected References: Definition of Death in Jewish Law**

Bleich, J.D. "Establishing Criteria of Death." In *Jewish Bioethics*, edited by F. Rosner and J.D. Bleich. New York: Hebrew Publishing Co., 1979.

Bleich, J.D. "Neurological Death and Time of Death Statutes" in *Jewish Bioethics,* edited by F. Rosner and J.D. Bleich. New York: Hebrew Publishing Co., 1979.

Bleich, J.D. *Judaism and Healing: Halachic Perspectives*. New York: Ktav Publishing, 1981.

Bleich, J.D. *Contemporary Halakhic Problems* (Vol I, III, IV). New York: Ktav Publishing & Yeshiva University Press, 1977, 1989, 1995.

Dorff, E.N. *Matters of Life and Death: A Jewish Approach to Modern Medical Ethics.* Philadelphia: Jewish Publication Society, 1998.

Goldfarb, D.C. " The Definition of Death." *Conservative Judaism* 30 (1976):10-22.

Jakobovits, I. *Jewish Medical Ethics*. New York: Bloch Publishing, 1974.

Rosner, F. *Modern Medicine and Jewish Ethics*. New York: Ktav Publishing, 1991.

Siegel, S. "Updating the Criteria of Death." *Conservative Judaism* 30 (1976):10-22.

Soloveichik, A. "The Halachic Definition of Death." In *Jewish Bioethics*, edited by F. Rosner and J.D. Bleich. New York: Hebrew Publishing Co., 1979.

Steinberg, A. "The Definition of Death" in *Medicine and Jewish Law (I),* edited by F. Rosner. Northvale, N.J.: Jason Aronson, Inc., 1991.

Tendler, M.D. *Responsa of Rabbi Moshe Feinstein: Critical Illness* (Vol 1). New York: Ktav Publishing, 1996.

**Selected References: Permissibility and Obligation for Cadaver Organ Donation**

Bleich, J.D. "Establishing Criteria of Death" in *Jewish Bioethics*, edited by F. Rosner and J.D. Bleich. New York: Hebrew Publishing Co., 1979.

Bleich, J.D. "Neurological Death and Time of Death Statutes" in *Jewish Bioethics,* edited by F. Rosner and J.D. Bleich. New York: Hebrew Publishing Co., 1979.

Bleich, J.D. *Judaism and Healing: Halachic Perspectives*. New York: Ktav Publishing, 1981.

Bleich, J.D. *Contemporary Halakhic Problems* (Vol I, III, IV). New York: Ktav Publishing & Yeshiva University Press, 1977, 1989, 1995.

Dorff, E.N. *Matters of Life and Death: A Jewish Approach to Modern Medical Ethics.* Philadelphia: Jewish Publication Society, 1998.

Jakobovits, I. *Jewish Medical Ethics*. New York: Bloch Publishing, 1974.

Rabinovitch, N.L. "What is Halachah for Organ Transplants?" in *Jewish Bioethics,* edited by F. Rosner and J.D. Bleich. New York: Hebrew Publishing Co., 1979.

Rosner, F. "Organ Transplantation in Jewish Law" in *Jewish Bioethics*, edited by F. Rosner and J.D. Bleich. New York: Hebrew Publishing Co., 1979.

Rosner, F. *Modern Medicine and Jewish Ethics*. New York: Ktav Publishing, 1991.

Soloveichik, A. "The Halachic Definition of Death" in *Jewish Bioethics*, edited by F. Rosner and J.D. Bleich. New York: Hebrew Publishing Co., 1979.

Steinberg, A. "The Definition of Death." In *Medicine and Jewish Law* (I), edited by F. Rosner. Northvale, N.J.: Jason Aronson, Inc., 1991.

Tendler, M.D. *Responsa of Rabbi Moshe Feinstein: Critical Illness* (Vol 1). New York: Ktav Publishing, 1996.

**Selected References: Cosmetic and Elective Surgery**

Bleich, J.D. *Contemporary Halakhic Problems* (Vol I). New York: Ktav Publishing & Yeshiva University Press, 1977.

Bleich, J.D. *Judaism and Healing: Halachic Perspectives*. New York: Ktav Publishing, 1981.

Dorff, E.N. *Matters of Life and Death: A Jewish Approach to Modern Medical Ethics.* Philadelphia: Jewish Publication Society, 1998.

Jakobovits, I. *Jewish Medical Ethics.* New York: Bloch Publishing, 1974.

Rosner, F. *Modern Medicine and Jewish Ethics.* New York: Ktav Publishing, 1991.

**Selected References: Confidentiality and Truth Telling**

Bleich, J.D. *Judaism and Healing: Halachic Perspectives.* New York: Ktav Publishing, 1981.

Bleich, J.D. "A Physician's Obligation with Regard to Disclosure of Information" in *Medicine and Jewish Law* (I), edited by F. Rosner. Northvale, N.J.: Jason Aronson, Inc., 1991.

Jakobovits I. *Jewish Medical Ethics.* New York: Bloch Publishing, 1974.

Rosner, F. "Medical Confidentiality in Judaism." *J. Halacha and Contemporary Society* XXXIII (1997): 5-16.

# Chapter 6: ISSUES OF PROCREATION AND ABORTION

## Selected References: Jewish Attitude Toward Sex and Sexuality

Dorff, E.N. "This is my Beloved, This is My Friend": A Rabbinic Letter on Intimate Relations. *Rabbinical Assembly*, 1996.

Dorff, E.N. *Matters of Life and Death: A Jewish Approach to Modern Medical Ethics.* Philadelphia: Jewish Publication Society, 1998.

Feldman, D.M. *Marital Relations, Birth Control and Abortion in Jewish Law.* (3rd ed.), New York: New York University Press, 1995.

Gold, M. *and Hannah Wept: Infertility, Adoption and the Jewish Couple.* Philadelphia: Jewish Publication Society, 1988. \

Gold, M. *Does God Belong in the Bedroom?* Philadelphia: Jewish Publication Society, 1992.

Grazi, R,V. *Be Fruitful and Multiply: Fertility Therapy and the Jewish Tradition.* Jerusalem: Genesis Jerusalem Press, 1994.

Jacob, W, and Zemer, M. *Fetus and Fertility in Jewish Law: Essays and Responsa.* Pittsburgh: Freehof Institute of Progressive Halachah, 1995.

Jakobovits, I. *Jewish Medical Ethics.* New York: Bloch Publishing, 1974.

Kimmelman, R. "Homosexuality and Family Centered Judaism." *Tikkun* 9 (1994): 4.

Novak, D. "Some Aspects of Sex, Society, and God in Judaism" in *Contemporary Jewish Ethics and Morality: A Reader*, edited by E.N. Dorff and L.E. Newman. New York: Oxford University Press, 1995.

Rosner, F. *Modern Medicine and Jewish Ethics.* New York: Ktav Publishing, 1991.

Shapiro, D.S. "Be Fruitful and Multiply" in *Jewish Bioethics*, edited by F. Rosner and J.D. Bleich. New York: Hebrew Publishing Co., 1979.

Waskow, A. "Down-to-Earth Judaism: Sexuality" in *Contemporary Jewish Ethics and Morality: A Reader*, edited by E.N. Dorff and L.E. Newman. New York: Oxford University Press, 1995.

**Selected References: The Obligation for Procreation**

Dorff, E.N. *Matters of Life and Death: A Jewish Approach to Modern Medical Ethics.* Philadelphia: Jewish Publication Society, 1998.

Feldman, D.M. *Marital Relations, Birth Control and Abortion in Jewish Law* (3rd ed.). New York: New York University Press, NY, 1995.

Gold, M. *and Hannah Wept: Infertility, Adoption and the Jewish Couple.* Philadelphia: Jewish Publication Society, 1988.

Gold, M. *Does God Belong in the Bedroom?* Philadelphia: Jewish Publication Society, 1992.

Grazi, R.V. *Be Fruitful and Multiply: Fertility Therapy and the Jewish Tradition.* Jerusalem: Genesis Jerusalem Press, 1994.

Jacob, W. and Zemer, M. *Fetus and Fertility in Jewish Law: Essays and Responsa.* Pittsburgh: Freehof Institute of Progressive Halachah, 1995.

Jakobovits, I. *Jewish Medical Ethics.* New York: Bloch Publishing, 1974.

Novak, D. "Some Aspects of Sex, Society, and God in Judaism" in *Contemporary Jewish Ethics and Morality: A Reader,* edited by E.N. Dorff and L.E. Newman. New York: Oxford University Press, 1995.

Rosner, F. *Modern Medicine and Jewish Ethics*. New York: Ktav Publishing, 1991.

Schachter, H. "Halachic Aspects of Family Planning." *J. Halacha and Contemporary Society* I (1982): 5-31.

Shapiro, D.S. "Be Fruitful and Multiply" in *Jewish Bioethics*, edited by F. Rosner and J.D. Bleich. New York: Hebrew Publishing Co., 1979.

Waskow, A. "Down-to-Earth Judaism: Sexuality" in *Contemporary Jewish Ethics and Morality: A Reader*, edited by E.N. Dorff and L.E. Newman. New York: Oxford University Press, 1995.

**Selected References: Genetic Counseling and Screening**

Abelson, K. "Prenatal Testing and Abortion." In *Proceedings of the Committee on Jewish Law and Standards of the Conservative Movement 1980-1985,* edited by D. Golinkin. Jerusalem: The Rabbinical Assembly and Institute of Applied Halachah, 1997.

Bleich, J.D. *Judaism and Healing: Halachic Perspectives*. New York: Ktav Publishing, 1981.

Bleich, J.D. *Contemporary Halakhic Problems* (Vol I). New York: Ktav Publishing & Yeshiva University Press, 1977, 1981, 1989, 1995.

Dorff, E.N. *Matters of Life and Death: A Jewish Approach to Modern Medical Ethics.* Philadelphia: Jewish Publication Society, 1998.

Feldman, D.M. *Marital Relations, Birth Control and Abortion in Jewish Law* (3rd ed.). New York: New York University Press, 1995.

Gold, M. *and Hannah Wept: Infertility, Adoption and the Jewish Couple.* Philadelphia: Jewish Publication Society, 1988.

Gold, M. *Does God Belong in the Bedroom?* Philadelphia: Jewish Publication Society, 1992.

Grazi, R.V. *Be Fruitful and Multiply: Fertility Therapy and the Jewish Tradition*. Jerusalem: Genesis Jerusalem Press, 1994.

Halperin, M. "Modern Perspectives on Halachah and Medicine" in *Medicine and Jewish Law* (I), edited by F. Rosner. Northvale, N.J.: Jason Aronson, Inc., 1991.

Jacob, W. and Zemer, M. *Fetus and Fertility in Jewish Law: Essays and Responsa.* Pittsburgh: Freehof Institute of Progressive Halachah, 1995.

Jakobovits, I. *Jewish Medical Ethics.* New York: Bloch Publishing, 1974.

Rosner, F. "Tay-Sachs Disease: To Screen or Not to Screen" in *Jewish Bioethics,* edited by F. Rosner and J.D. Bleich. New York: Hebrew Publishing Co., 1979.

Rosner, F. *Modern Medicine and Jewish Ethics.* New York: Ktav Publishing, 1991.

Rosner, F. "Rabbi Moshe Feinstein's Influence on Medical Halachah" in *Medicine and Jewish Law* (II), edited by F. Rosner. Northvale, N.J.: Jason Aronson, Inc., 1993.

Rosner, F. and Tendler, M.D. *Practical Medical Halachah.* Northvale, N.J.: Jason Aronson, Inc., 1997.

Rosner, F. *Pioneers in Jewish Medical Ethics.* Northvale, N.J.: Jason Aronson, Inc., 1998.

Schachter, H. "Halachic Aspects of Family Planning." *J Halacha and Contemporary Society* I (1982): 5-31.

**Selected References: Contraception**

Bleich, J.D. *Contemporary Halakhic Problems* (Vol I). New York: Ktav Publishing and Yeshiva University Press, 1977.

Bleich, J.D. *Judaism and Healing: Halachic Perspectives.* New York: Ktav Publishing, 1981.

Dorff, E.N. *Matters of Life and Death: A Jewish Approach to Modern Medical Ethics.* Philadelphia: Jewish Publication Society, 1998.

Feldman, D.M. *Marital Relations, Birth Control and Abortion in Jewish Law* (3rd ed.). New York: New York University Press, 1995.

Gold, M. *and Hannah Wept: Infertility, Adoption and the Jewish Couple.* Philadelphia: Jewish Publication Society, 1988.

Gold, M. *Does God Belong in the Bedroom?* Philadelphia: Jewish Publication Society, 1992.

Grazi, R.V. *Be Fruitful and Multiply: Fertility Therapy and the Jewish Tradition.* Jerusalem: Genesis Jerusalem Press, 1994.

Jacob, W. and Zemer, M. *Fetus and Fertility in Jewish Law: Essays and Responsa.* Pittsburgh: Freehof Institute of Progressive Halachah, 1995.

Jakobovits, I. *Jewish Medical Ethics*. New York: Bloch Publishing, 1974.

Rosner, F. "Contraception." In *Jewish Bioethics*, edited by F. Rosner and J.D. Bleich. New York: Hebrew Publishing Co., 1979.

Rosner, F. *Modern Medicine and Jewish Ethics*. New York: Ktav Publishing, 1991.

Rosner, F. and Tendler, M.D. *Practical Medical Halachah*. Northvale, N.J.: Jason Aronson, Inc., 1997.

Rosner, F. *Pioneers in Jewish Medical Ethics*. Northvale, N.J.: Jason Aronson, Inc., 1998.

Schachter, H. "Halachic Aspects of Family Planning." *J. Halacha and Contemporary Society* I (1982): 5-31.

Tendler, M.D. "Contraception and Abortion" in *Medicine and Jewish Law* (I), edited by F. Rosner. Northvale, N.J.: Jason Aronson, Inc., 1991.

**Selected References: Adoption**

Dorff, E.N. *Matters of Life and Death: A Jewish Approach to Modern Medical Ethics*. Philadelphia: Jewish Publication Society, 1998.

Feldman, D.M. *Marital Relations, Birth Control and Abortion in Jewish Law* (3rd ed.). New York: New York University Press, 1995.

Gold, M. *and Hannah Wept: Infertility, Adoption and the Jewish Couple.* Philadelphia: Jewish Publication Society, 1988.

Gold, M. *Does God Belong in the Bedroom?* Philadelphia: Jewish Publication Society, 1992.

Grazi, R.V. *Be Fruitful and Multiply: Fertility Therapy and the Jewish Tradition.* Jerusalem: Genesis Jerusalem Press, 1994.

Jacob, W. and Zemer, M. *Fetus and Fertility in Jewish Law: Essays and Responsa.* Pittsburgh: Freehof Institute of Progressive Halachah, 1995.

Jakobovits, I. *Jewish Medical Ethics.* New York: Bloch Publishing, 1974.

Schachter, M. "Various Aspects of Adoption." *J. Halacha and Contemporary Society* IV (1982): 93-115.

**Selected References: Infertility Treatment - Advanced Reproductive Technology**

Bleich, J.D. "Test-Tube Babies" in *Jewish Bioethics*, edited by F. Rosner and J.D. Bleich. New York: Hebrew Publishing Co., 1979.

Bleich, J.D. *Judaism and Healing: Halachic Perspectives*. New York: Ktav Publishing, 1981.

Bleich, J.D. *Contemporary Halakhic Problems* (Vol I,IV). New York: Ktav Publishing and Yeshiva University Press, 1977, 1981, 1989, 1995.

Bleich, J.D. "Sperm Banking in Anticipation of Infertility." *Tradition* 29 (1995): 4.

Cohen, A.S. "Artificial Insemination." *J. Halacha and Contemporary Society* XIII (1987): 43-60.

Dorff, E.N. "Artificial Insemination, Egg Donation and Adoption." *Conservative Judaism* 49 (1996): 3-60.

Dorff, E.N. *Matters of Life and Death: A Jewish Approach to Modern Medical Ethics*. Philadelphia: Jewish Publication Society, 1998.

Feld, E. "Technology and Halachah: The Use of Artificial Insemination." *Conservative Judaism* 48 (1996): 49-56.

Feldman, D.M. *Marital Relations, Birth Control and Abortion in Jewish Law* (3rd ed.). New York: New York University Press, 1995.

Gold, M. *and Hannah Wept: Infertility, Adoption and the Jewish Couple.* Philadelphia: Jewish Publication Society, 1988.

Gold, M. *Does God Belong in the Bedroom?* Philadelphia: Jewish Publication Society, 1992.

Grazi, R.V. *Be Fruitful and Multiply: Fertility Therapy and the Jewish Tradition.* Jerusalem: Genesis Jerusalem Press, 1994.

Green, J. "Artificial Insemination in Israel." *Jewish Medical Ethics* II:1 (1991): 21-28.

Halperin, M. "In-Vitro Fertilization, Embryo Transfer and Embryo Freezing." *Jewish Medical Ethics* I:1 (1988): 25-30.

Jacob, W. and Zemer, M. *Fetus and Fertility in Jewish Law: Essays and Responsa.* Pittsburgh: Freehof Institute of Progressive Halachah, 1995.

Jakobovits, I. *Jewish Medical Ethics.* New York: Bloch Publishing, 1974.

Jakobovits, I. "Male Infertility: Halachic Issues in Investigation and Management." *Tradition* 27 (1993): 4-21.

Rosenfeld, A. "Generation, Gestation, and Judaism." *Tradition* 12 (1971): 78-87.

Rosner, F. "Artificial Insemination in Jewish Law" in *Jewish Bioethics*, edited by F. Rosner and J.D. Bleich. New York: Hebrew Publishing Co., 1979.

Rosner, F. *Modern Medicine and Jewish Ethics*. New York: Ktav Publishing, 1991.

Rosner, F. and Tendler, M.D. *Practical Medical Halachah*. Northvale, N.J.: Jason Aronson, Inc., 1997.

Rosner, F. *Pioneers in Jewish Medical Ethics*. Northvale, N.J.: Jason Aronson, Inc., 1998.

**Selected References: Infertility Treatment - Surrogate Motherhood**

Bleich, J.D. *Contemporary Halakhic Problems* (Vol I). New York: Ktav Publishing and Yeshiva University Press, 1977.

Bleich, J.D. "In Vitro Fertilization: Questions of Maternal Identity and Conversion." *Tradition* 25 (1991): 82-102.

Bleich, J.D. Surrogate Motherhood. *Tradition* 32 (1998): 146-167.

Clark, E.D., Silverman, Z., "Surrogate Motherhood in the Case of High-Risk Pregnancy." *J. Halacha and Contemporary Society* 38 (1999): 5-38.

Dorff, E.N. *Matters of Life and Death: A Jewish Approach to Modern Medical Ethics.* Philadelphia: Jewish Publication Society, 1998.

Feldman, D.M. *Marital Relations, Birth Control and Abortion in Jewish Law* (3rd ed.). New York: New York University Press, 1995.

Gold, M. *and Hannah Wept: Infertility, Adoption and the Jewish Couple.* Philadelphia: Jewish Publication Society, 1988.

Gold, M. *Does God Belong in the Bedroom?* Philadelphia: Jewish Publication Society, 1992.

Grazi, R.V. *Be Fruitful and Multiply: Fertility Therapy and the Jewish Tradition.* Jerusalem: Genesis Jerusalem Press, 1994.

Jacob, W. and Zemer, M. *Fetus and Fertility in Jewish Law: Essays and Responsa.* Pittsburgh: Freehof Institute of Progressive Halachah, 1995.

Rosenfeld, A. "Generation, Gestation, and Judaism." *Tradition* 12 (1971): 78-87.

Rosner, F. *Modern Medicine and Jewish Ethics*. New York: Ktav Publishing, 1991.

Segal, L. "Surrogacy: The British Community Wrestles with a Controversial Issue." *Amit* (Spring 1998): 17-20.

**Selected References: Infertility Treatment – Cloning**

Bleich, J.D. "Cloning: Homologous Reproduction and Jewish Law." *Tradition* 32 (1998): 47-86.

Broyde, M. "Cloning People and Jewish Law: A Preliminary Analysis." *J. Halacha and Contemporary Society* 34 (1997): 23-65.

Dorff, E.N. *Matters of Life and Death: A Jewish Approach to Modern Medical Ethics.* Philadelphia: Jewish Publication Society, 1998.

Grazi, R.V. and Wolowelsky, J.B. "On Cloning." *Amit* (Summer 1998): 6-9.

Loike, J.D. and Steinberg, A. "Human Cloning and Halachic Perspectives." *Tradition* 32 (1998): 31-46.

Rosenfeld, A. "Generation, Gestation, and Judaism." *Tradition* 12 (1971): 78-87.

**Selected References: Sex Preference and Selection**

Bleich, J.D. *Judaism and Healing: Halachic Perspectives.* New York: Ktav Publishing, 1981.

Dorff, E.N. *Matters of Life and Death: A Jewish Approach to Modern Medical Ethics.* Philadelphia: Jewish Publication Society, 1998.

Feldman, D.M. *Marital Relations, Birth Control and Abortion in Jewish Law* (3rd ed.). New York: New York University Press, 1995.

Gold, M. *and Hannah Wept: Infertility, Adoption and the Jewish Couple.* Philadelphia: Jewish Publication Society, 1988.

Gold, M. *Does God Belong in the Bedroom?* Philadelphia: Jewish Publication Society, 1992.

Grazi, R.V. *Be Fruitful and Multiply: Fertility Therapy and the Jewish Tradition.* Jerusalem: Genesis Jerusalem Press, 1994.

Jacob, W. and Zemer, M. *Fetus and Fertility in Jewish Law: Essays and Responsa.* Pittsburgh: Freehof Institute of Progressive Halachah, 1995.

Jakobovits, I. *Jewish Medical Ethics.* New York: Bloch Publishing, 1974.

Rosner, F. *Modern Medicine and Jewish Ethics.* New York: Ktav Publishing, 1991.

Rosner, F. and Tendler, M.D. *Practical Medical Halachah.* Northvale, N.J.: Jason Aronson, Inc., 1997.

Rosner, F. *Pioneers in Jewish Medical Ethics*. Northvale, N.J.: Jason Aronson, Inc., 1998.

**Selected References: Multi-Gestational Pregnancy Reduction**

Bleich, J.D. *Judaism and Healing: Halachic Perspectives.* New York: Ktav Publishing, 1981.

Dorff, E.N. *Matters of Life and Death: A Jewish Approach to Modern Medical Ethics.* Philadelphia: Jewish Publication Society, 1998.

Feldman, D.M. *Marital Relations, Birth Control and Abortion in Jewish Law* (3rd ed.), New York: New York University Press, 1995.

Gold, M. *and Hannah Wept: Infertility, Adoption and the Jewish Couple.* Philadelphia: Jewish Publication Society, 1988.

Gold, M. *Does God Belong in the Bedroom?* Philadelphia: Jewish Publication Society, 1992.

Grazi, R.V. *Be Fruitful and Multiply: Fertility Therapy and the Jewish Tradition.* Jerusalem: Genesis Jerusalem Press, 1994.

Jacob, W. and Zemer, M. *Fetus and Fertility in Jewish Law: Essays and Responsa.* Pittsburgh: Freehof Institute of Progressive Halachah, 1995.

Jakobovits, I. *Jewish Medical Ethics.* New York: Bloch Publishing, 1974.

Mehlman, Y. "Multi-Fetal Pregnancy Reduction." *J. Halacha and Contemporary Society* XXVII (1994): 35-68.

Rosner, F. *Modern Medicine and Jewish Ethics.* New York: Ktav Publishing, 1991.

Rosner, F. and Tendler, M.D. *Practical Medical Halachah.* Northvale, N.J.: Jason Aronson, Inc., 1997.

Rosner, F. *Pioneers in Jewish Medical Ethics.* Northvale, N.J.: Jason Aronson, Inc., 1998.

Rudman, Z.C. "Fetal Rights and Maternal Obligations." *J. Halacha and Contemporary Society* XIII (1987): 113-124.

**Selected References: Abortion**

Abelson, K. "Prenatal Testing and Abortion." In *Proceedings of the Committee on Jewish Law and Standards of the Conservative Movement 1980-1985*, edited by D. Golinkin. Jerusalem: The Rabbinical Assembly and Institute of Applied Halachah, 1997.

Bleich, J.D. "Abortion in Halachic Literature" in *Jewish Bioethics*, edited by F. Rosner and J.D. Bleich. New York: Hebrew Publishing Co., 1979.

Bleich, J.D. *Judaism and Healing: Halachic Perspectives*. New York: Ktav Publishing, 1981.

Bleich, J.D. *Contemporary Halakhic Problems* (Vol IV). New York: Ktav Publishing and Yeshiva University Press, 1995.

Bokser, B.Z. and Abeslon, K. "A Statement on the Permissibility of Abortion." In *Proceedings of the Committee on Jewish Law and Standards of the Conservative Movement 1980-1985,* edited by D. Golinkin. Jerusalem: The Rabbinical Assembly and Institute of Applied Halachah, 1997.

Dorff, E.N. *Matters of Life and Death: A Jewish Approach to Modern Medical Ethics.* Philadelphia: Jewish Publication Society, 1998.

Feldman, D.L. "Abortion: The Jewish View." In *Proceedings of the Committee on Jewish Law and Standards of the Conservative Movement 1980-1985,* edited by D. Golinkin. Jerusalem: The Rabbinical Assembly and Institute of Applied Halachah, 1997.

Feldman, D.M. *Marital Relations, Birth Control and Abortion in Jewish Law* (3rd ed.). New York: New York University Press, 1995.

Feldman, D.M. "On This Matter of Abortion" in *Contemporary Jewish Ethics and Morality: A Reader,* edited by E.N. Dorff and L.E. Newman. New York: Oxford University Press, 1995.

Gold, M. *and Hannah Wept: Infertility, Adoption and the Jewish Couple.* Philadelphia: Jewish Publication Society, 1988.

Gold, M. *Does God Belong in the Bedroom?* Philadelphia: Jewish Publication Society, 1992.

Gordis, R. "Abortion: Major Wrong or Basic Right?" In *Proceedings of the Committee on Jewish Law and Standards of the Conservative Movement 1980-1985,* edited by D. Golinkin. Jerusalem: The Rabbinical Assembly and Institute of Applied Halachah, 1997.

Grazi, R.V. *Be Fruitful and Multiply: Fertility Therapy and the Jewish Tradition.* Jerusalem: Genesis Jerusalem Press, 1994.

Jacob, W. and Zemer, M. *Fetus and Fertility in Jewish Law: Essays and Responsa.* Pittsburgh: Freehof Institute of Progressive Halachah, 1995.

Jakobovits, I. *Jewish Medical Ethics.* New York: Bloch Publishing, 1974.

Jakobovits, I. "Jewish Views on Abortion." In *Jewish Bioethics*, edited by F. Rosner and J.D. Bleich. New York: Hebrew Publishing Co., 1979.

Kirschner, R. "The Halachic Status of the Fetus with Respect to Abortion." *Conservative Judaism* 34 (1981):3-16.

Klein, I. "A Teshuvah on Abortion." In *Proceedings of the Committee on Jewish Law and Standards of the Conservative Movement 1980-1985,* edited by D. Golinkin. Jerusalem: The Rabbinical Assembly and Institute of Applied Halachah, 1997.

Lubansky, S.B. "Judaism and Justification of Abortion for Nonmedical Reasons." In *Contemporary Jewish Ethics and Morality: A Reader,* edited by E.N. Dorff and L.E. Newman. New York: Oxford University Press, 1995.

Rosner, F. *Modern Medicine and Jewish Ethics.* New York: Ktav Publishing, 1991.

Rosner, F. and Tendler, M.D. *Practical Medical Halachah.* Northvale, N.J.: Jason Aronson, Inc., 1997.

Rosner, F. *Pioneers in Jewish Medical Ethics.* Northvale, N.J.: Jason Aronson, Inc., 1998.

Tendler, M.D. "Contraception and Abortion" in *Medicine and Jewish Law* (I), edited by F. Rosner. Northvale, N.J.: Jason Aronson, Inc., 1991.

## Chapter 7: END OF LIFE ISSUES

### Selected References: Advance Directives

Dorff, E.N. *Matters of Life and Death: A Jewish Approach to Modern Medical Ethics.* Philadelphia: Jewish Publication Society, 1998.

Ifrah, A.J. "The Living Will." *J. Halacha and Contemporary Society* XXIV (1992): 121-152

Schwartz, R.A. "The Power to Choose: Why Jews Are Signing Living Wills." *The Jewish Monthly* (May 1994): 36-46.

**Selected References: Withdrawing and Withholding Treatment in the Face of Pain and Suffering**

Abraham, A.S. "Euthanasia" in *Medicine and Jewish Law* (I) edited by F. Rosner. Northvale, N.J.: Jason Aronson, Inc., 1991.

Abraham, A.S. "The Goses" in *Medicine and Jewish Law* (II), edited by F. Rosner. Northvale, N.J.: Jason Aronson, Inc., 1993.

Bleich, J.D. "The Quinlan Case: A Jewish Perspective" in *Jewish Bioethics,* edited by F. Rosner and J.D. Bleich. New York: Hebrew Publishing Co., 1979.

Bleich, J.D. *Judaism and Healing: Halachic Perspectives*. New York: Ktav Publishing, 1981.

Bleich, J.D. *Contemporary Halakhic Problems* (Vol I-IV). New York: Ktav Publishing and Yeshiva University Press, 1977, 1981, 1989, 1995.

Bleich, J.D. "The Treatment of the Terminally Ill." *Tradition* 30 (1996): 51-87.

Cohen, A. "Whose Body? Living with Pain." *J. Halacha and Contemporary Society*, XXXII (1996):39-64.

Dorff, E.N. "Rabbi, I'm Dying." *Conservative Judaism* 37 (1984): 3751.

Dorff, E.N. "A Jewish Approach to End-Stage Medical Care." *Conservative Judaism* 43 (1991): 3-51.

Dorff, E.N. *Matters of Life and Death: A Jewish Approach to Modern Medical Ethics.* Philadelphia: Jewish Publication Society, 1998.

Dorff, E.N. "Teshuvah on Assisted Suicide." *Conservative Judaism* 50 (1998): 3-24.

Eilberg, A. "On Halachic Approaches to Medical Care for the Terminally Ill: A Response." *Conservative Judaism* 43 (1991): 92-94.

Friedman, F. "The Chronic Vegetative Patient: A Torah Perspective." *J. Halacha and Contemporary Society* XXVI (1994): 88-109.

Friedman, Y. "Defining a Goses" in *Medicine and Jewish Law* (II), edited by F. Rosner. Northvale, N.J.: Jason Aronson, Inc., 1993.

Herring, B.F. *Jewish Ethics and Halachah for Our Time*. New York: Yeshiva University Press, 1984.

Jakobovits, I. *Jewish Medical Ethics*. New York: Bloch Publishing, 1974.

Koenigsberg, M. *Halachah and Medicine Today*. New York: Feldheim Publishers, 1997.

Nevins, M.A. "No Heroics – A Jewish Perspective on Artificial Feeding of the Dying." *J. Med. Soc. N.J.* 77 (1980): 442-444.

Prouser, J.H. "Being of Sound Mind and Judgement: Rethinking Sanctions in the Case of Physician Assisted Suicide." *Conservative Judaism* 49 (1997): 3-16.

Reisner, A.I. "A Halachic Ethic of Care for the Terminally Ill." *Conservative Judaism* 43 (1991): 52-94.

Rosner, F. "The Jewish Attitude Toward Euthanasia" in *Jewish Bioethics*, edited by F. Rosner and J.D. Bleich. New York: Hebrew Publishing Co., 1979.

Rosner, F. *Modern Medicine and Jewish Ethics*. New York: Ktav Publishing, 1991.

Rosner, F. "Euthanasia" in *Contemporary Jewish Ethics and Morality: A Reader,* edited by E.N. Dorff and L.E. Newman. New York: Oxford University Press, 1995.

Rosner, F. *Pioneers in Jewish Medical Ethics*. Northvale, N.J.: Jason Aronson, Inc., 1998.

Roth, J. "On Halachic Approaches to Medical Care for the Terminally Ill: A Response." *Conservative Judaism* 43 (1991):95-96.

Schohet, D.M. "Mercy Death in Jewish Law." *Conservative Judaism* 8 (1952): 1-15.

Schostak, Z. "Ethical Guidelines for Treatment of the Dying Patient." *J. Halacha and Contemporary Society* XXII (1991):62-86.

Sherwin, B. "A View of Euthanasia" in *Contemporary Jewish Ethics and Morality: A Reader*, edited by E.N. Dorff and L.E. Newman. New York: Oxford University Press, 1995.

Tendler, M.D. *Responsa of Rav Moshe Feinstein: Critical Illness* (Vol 1). New York: Ktav Publishing, 1996.

Tendler, M.D. and Rosner, F. "Quality and Sanctity of Life in the Talmud and the Midrash." *Tradition* 28 (1993):18-27.

**Selected References: Autopsy**

Bleich, J.D. *Contemporary Halakhic Problems* (Vol I). New York: Ktav Publishing and Yeshiva University Press,1977.

Bleich, J.D. *Judaism and Healing: Halachic Perspectives*. New York: Ktav Publishing, 1981.

Dorff, E.N. *Matters of Life and Death: A Jewish Approach to Modern Medical Ethics.* Philadelphia: Jewish Publication Society, 1998.

Herring, B.F. *Jewish Ethics and Halachah for Our Time*. New York: Yeshiva University Press, 1984.

Jakobovits, I. *Jewish Medical Ethics*. New York: Bloch Publishing, 1974.

Rosner, F. "Autopsy in Jewish Law" in *Jewish Bioethics,* edited by F. Rosner and J.D. Bleich. New York: Hebrew Publishing Co., 1979.

Rosner, F. *Modern Medicine and Jewish Ethics*. New York: Ktav Publishing, 1991.

Shohet, D.M. "Post Mortem Examination for Medical Purposes in Jewish Law." *Proceedings of the Committee on Jewish Law and Standards of the Conservative Movement, 1927-1970.*

**Selected References: Medical Malpractice and Physician Fees**

Dorff, E.N. *Matters of Life and Death: A Jewish Approach to Modern Medical Ethics.* Philadelphia: Jewish Publication Society, 1998.

Jakobovits, I. *Jewish Medical Ethics.* New York: Bloch Publishing, 1974.

Kottek, S. "The Practice of Medicine in the Bible and Talmud" in *Pioneers in Jewish Medical Ethics*, edited by F. Rosner. Northvale, N.J.: Jason Aronson, Inc., 1998.

Rosner, F. "The Physician and the Patient in Jewish Law" in *Jewish Bioethics*, edited by F. Rosner and J.D. Bleich. New York: Hebrew Publishing Co., 1979.

Rosner, F. *Modern Medicine and Jewish Ethics.* New York: Ktav Publishing, 1991.

## BIBLIOGRAPHY AND SUGGESTED READING

### Books (English)

Abraham, A.S. *Comprehensive Guide to Medical Halachah.* New York: Feldheim Publishers, 1990.

Barcalow, E. *Moral Philosophy: Theory and Issues*. Belmont, Ca.: Wadsworth Publishing Co., 1994.

Barron, J.L. *A Treasury of Jewish Quotations*. Northvale, N.J.: Jason Aronson, Inc., 1996.

Beauchamp, T.L. and Childress, J.F. *Principles of Biomedical Ethics* (2nd ed.). New York: Oxford University Press, 1994.

Berkovits, E. *Faith After the Holocaust*. New York: Ktav Publishing, 1973.

Bleich, J.D. *Judaism and Healing: Halachic Perspectives*. New York: Ktav Publishing, 1981.

Bleich, J.D. *Contemporary Halakhic Problems* (Vol I-IV). New York: Ktav Publishing and Yeshiva University Press, 1977, 1981, 1989, 1995.

Borowitz, E.B. *Reform Jewish Ethics and the Halakhah: An Experiment in Decision-making*. West Orange, N.J.: Behrman House, Inc., 1994.

Bulka, R.P. *Judaism on Illness and Suffering*. Northvale, N.J.: Jason Aronson, Inc. 1998.

Cohen, A.A. and Mendes-Flohr, P. (Eds). *Contemporary Jewish Religious Thought.* New York: Free Press, 1977.

Dorff, E.N. *Conservative Judaism: Our Ancestors to Our Descendants*. New York: United Synagogue of America, 1977.

Dorff E.N. and Newman, L.E. (Eds). *Contemporary Jewish Ethics and Morality: A Reader*. New York: Oxford University Press, 1995.

Dorff, E.N. *Matters of Life and Death: A Jewish Approach to Modern Medical Ethics.* Philadelphia: Jewish Publication Society, 1998.

Elon, M. *"The Principles of Jewish Law"* (Encyclopedia Judaica). Jerusalem: Keter Publishing House, 1994.

Feldman, D.M. *Marital Relations, Birth Control and Abortion in Jewish Law* (3rd ed.). New York: New York University Press, 1995.

Freehof, S.B. *Modern Reform Responsa.* Cincinnati: Hebrew Union College Press, 1971.

Freehof, S.B. *Reform Responsa for Our Time*. Cincinnati: Hebrew Union College Press, 1977.

Freehof, S.B. *New Reform Responsa*. Cincinnati: Hebrew Union College Press, 1980.

Freehof, S.B. *Today's Reform Responsa*. Cincinnati: Hebrew Union College Press, 1990.

Gold, M. *and Hannah Wept: Infertility, Adoption and the Jewish Couple.* Philadelphia: Jewish Publication Society, 1988.

Gold, M. *Does God Belong in the Bedroom?* Philadelphia: Jewish Publication Society, 1992.

Golinkin, D. (Ed). *Proceedings of the Committee on Jewish Law and Standards of the Conservative Movement 1927-1970.* Jerusalem: The Rabbinical Assembly and Institute of Applied Halachah, 1997.

Golinkin, D. (Ed). *Proceedings of the Committee on Jewish Law and Standards of the Conservative Movement 1980-1985.* Jerusalem: The Rabbinical Assembly and Institute of Applied Halachah, 1997.

Grazi, R.V. *Be Fruitful and Multiply: Fertility Therapy and the Jewish Tradition.* Jerusalem: Genesis Jerusalem Press, 1994.

Herring, B.F. *Jewish Ethics and Halachah for Our Time*. New York: Yeshiva University Press, 1984.

Isaacs, R.H. *Judaism, Medicine and Healing*. Northvale, N.J.: Jason Aronson, Inc., 1998.

Jacob, W. *American Reform Responsa*. New York: Central Conference of American Rabbis, 1983.

Jacob, W. *Contemporary American Reform Responsa*. New York: Central Conference of American Rabbis, 1987.

Jacob, W. *Questions and Reform Jewish Answers: New American Reform Responsa*. New York: Central Conference of American Rabbis, 1992.

Jacob, W. and Zemer, M. *Fetus and Fertility in Jewish Law: Essays and Responsa*. Pittsburgh: Freehof Institute of Progressive Halachah, 1995.

Jacob, W. and Zemer, M. *Death and Euthanasia in Jewish Law: Essays and Responsa*. Pittsburgh: Freehof Institute of Progressive Halachah, 1995.

Jakobovits, I. *Jewish Medical Ethics*. New York: Bloch Publishing, 1974.

Koenigsberg, M. *Halachah and Medicine Today*. New York: Feldheim Publishers, 1997.

Kushner, H. *When Bad Things Happen to Good People.* New York: Schocken Press, 1981.

Landesman, D. *A Practical Guide to Torah Learning.* Northvale, N.J.: Jason Aronson, Inc., 1995.

Rosenthal, G.S. *The Many Faces of Judaism: Orthodox, Conservative, Reconstructionist and Reform.* West Orange, N.J.: Behrman House, Inc., 1978.

Rosner, F. and Bleich, J.D. (Eds). *Jewish Bioethics.* New York: Hebrew Publishing Co., 1979.

Rosner, F. *Modern Medicine and Jewish Ethics.* New York: Ktav Publishing, 1991.

Rosner F. (Ed). *Medicine and Jewish Law* (I and II). Northvale, N.J.: Jason Aronson, Inc., 1991, 1993.

Rosner, F. (translator). *Julius Preuss' Biblical and Talmudic Medicine.* Northvale, N.J.: Jason Aronson, Inc., 1993.

Rosner, F. and Kottek, S.S. (Eds). *Moses Maimonides: Physician, Scientist and Philosopher.* Northvale, N.J.: Jason Aronson, Inc., 1993.

Rosner, F. and Tendler, M.D. *Practical Medical Halachah.* Northvale, N.J.: Jason Aronson, Inc., 1997.

Rosner, F. *Pioneers in Jewish Medical Ethics*. Northvale, N.J.: Jason Aronson, Inc., 1998.

Sacks, J. *Arguments for the Sake of Heaven: Emerging Trends in Traditional Judaism*. Northvale, N.J.: Jason Aronson, Inc., 1991.

Slae, M. *Smoking and Damage to Health in the Halachah.* Jerusalem: Acharai Publications, 1990.

Telushkin, J. *Jewish Literacy.* New York: William Morrow and Co., 1991.

Tendler, M.D. *Responsa of Rav Moshe Feinstein: Critical Illness* (Vol 1). New York: Ktav Publishing, 1996.

Wurzburger, W.S. *Ethics of Responsibility: Pluralistic Approaches to Covenantal Ethics.* Philadelphia: Jewish Publication Society, 1994.

Zohar, N.J. *Alternatives in Jewish Bioethics*. Albany: State University of New York Press, 1997.

**Journals**

*Conservative Judaism*. New York: Jewish Theological Seminary

*Journal of Halachah and Contemporary Society*. Staten Island: Rabbi Jacob Joseph School.

*Proceedings of the Committee on Bio-ethics.* Philadelphia: Central Conference of American Rabbis

*Religious Traditions and Health Care Decisions Series.* Chicago: The Park Ridge Center

*Tradition: A Journal of Orthodox Jewish Thought.* New York: Rabbinical Council of America.

## GLOSSARY

**Achronim** – "the later ones" – later Biblical and Talmudic commentators after the publishing of the *Shulchan Aruch*

**Aggada** - non-legal discussions or stories offering moral and historical teachings and observations

**Amora** (*amoraim* – plural) – rabbis from the time of the Gemara

**Arba'ah Turim** (also known as Tur) - 14th-century code of Jewish law compiled by R. Jacob ben Asher. Divided into four sections which serve as the basis for all subsequent codes: *Orach Chayim*-- laws of prayers, Sabbath and festivals; *Yoreh Deah*-- laws of forbidden and permitted foods, vows and purity; *Even Haezer*-- laws of marriage, divorce and sexual relations; *Choshen Mishpat*-- civil and criminal law, inheritance and property

**Aruch HaShulchan** – 19th-century update of the *Shulchan Aruch* composed by R. Yechiel Epstein

**Autonomy** - self-determination, ability of an individual to decide issues for himself

**BCE** – Before Common Era, equivalent to BC

**Babylonian Talmud** – version of Talmud composed in Babylon. Written in Aramaic, consists of 35 tractates

**Bamidbar** – fourth book of the Pentateuch - *Numbers*

**Beneficence** – ideal of doing good for the benefit of another individual

**Biomedical Ethics** (bioethics) - subcategory of general ethics in which standard philosophical principles are applied in the analysis of moral problems and judgments as they specifically relate to clinical medicine, behavioral sciences and biomedical sciences

**B'reishit** – first book of the Pentateuch - *Genesis*

**CE** – Common Era, equivalent to AD

**Devarim** – fifth book of the Pentateuch - *Deuteronomy*

**Dina d'malchuta dina** – Hebrew expression meaning "the law of the land is the law"

**Ethics** - the branch of philosophy that studies moral values and judgments

**G'zeira** (*g'zeirot* – plural) – rabbinic decrees designed to prevent an action or "make a fence" around the Torah (prevent the violation of a Biblical commandment).

**Gaon** – head of a Babylon academy or yeshiva

**Gaonic period** - period of time following the redaction of the Talmud until the $10^{th}$ century

**Gemara** – extensive commentary on the Mishnah

**Halacha** – Hebrew term for Jewish law, literally: "the way"

**Iggrot Moshe** – published responsa of Rabbi Moshe Feinstein, zt"l

**Jerusalem Talmud** – version of Talmud composed in ancient Palestine, also known as Palestinian Talmud

**Justice** – ideal of equality

**Maimonides** – acronym for Rabbi Moses ben Maimon, also known as Rambam, revered $12^{th}$-century commentator, philosopher and physician

**Mappah** – ("Tablecloth") – contemporaneous gloss to the *Shulchan Aruch* by R. Moses Isserles (known as the Rama) that describes the practices of Ashkenazi (European) Jewry

**Mesorah** - religious heritage transmitted from Moses to successive generations

**Midrash** (*midrashim* – plural) – legal and homiletic commentaries on the Tanach composed between the $2^{nd}$ and $11^{th}$ centuries that fill in gaps in the story line and provide explanations of complexities

**Minhag** (*minhagim* – plural) – religious customs

**Mishnah** – First part of the Talmud, redacted by Rabbi Judah the Prince around 200 CE. Written in Hebrew, it consists of six major divisions called Sidrei (Orders), Zeraim - laws of agriculture, Moed - laws pertaining to the Sabbath and holidays, Nashim - laws pertaining to marriage, and divorce, Nezikin - civil laws and damages, Kodashim - sacrifices offered in the Temple, and Toharot - ritual purity.

**Mishnah B'rurah** – early $20^{th}$-century update of the *Shulchan Aruch* by Rabbi Israel Meir Kagan, who is also known as the Chafetz Chaim

**Mishneh Torah** – early code of Jewish law composed by Maimonides. Consist of 14 volumes, also known as Yad Chazakah

**Mitzvah** (*Mitzvot* – plural) – Hebrew word for Biblical commandment or religious obligation

**Nachmanides** – acronym for R. Moses ben Nachman, $13^{th}$-century commentator, philosopher and physician

**Nishmat Avraham** – authoritative contemporary work by Dr. A.S. Avraham on Jewish medical law containing many unpublished responsa by R. S.Z. Auerbach, zt"l

**Nonmaleficence** – ideal of not doing any harm to another individual

**Oral Law** – oral tradition (*Torah she'ba'al peh*), Talmud

**Perush** (*perushim* – plural) - elucidative commentaries on the Tanach, Talmud and codes of Jewish law

**Rashi** – acronym for R. Shlomo ben Yitzchak, the pre-eminent Biblical and Talmudic commentator who lived in the 11th century

**Responsum** (responsa – plural) – Rabbinic answers to questions (Hebrew – *t'shuvah, t'shuvot*)

**Rishonim** -the "first ones" – early Biblical and Talmudic commentators who lived before the publishing of the *Shulchan Aruch* (Code of Jewish Law)

**She'eilot** - questions submitted to rabbis

**Shmirat Shabbat K'hilchata** – authoritative contemporary text by R. Y. Neuwirth dealing with the laws of *Shabbat*

**Sh'mot** – second book of the Pentateuch - *Exodus*

**Shulchan Aruch** ("Set Table") – definitive Code of Jewish Law composed by R. Joseph Caro in the 16th century

**Takanah** (*Takanot* – plural) - rabbinic enactments that are usually designed to impose a duty to perform some act

**Talmud** – compilation of the Oral Law consisting of the Mishnah and Gemara

**Tana** (*Tannaim* – plural) – rabbis from the time of the Mishnah

**Tanach** – acronym for canonized Hebrew Bible or Old Testament, which is comprised of the Torah, the N'vi'im (Prophets) and K'tuvim (Writings)

**Torah** - Pentateuch, Five Books of Moses, Written Law (*Torah she'bichtav*)

**Tosafot** - a group of $12^{th-}$ and $13^{th}$-century commentators

**Tur** - see Arba'ah Turim

**Tzitz Eliezer** – published responsa of Rabbi Eliezer Waldenberg

**Vayikra** – third book of the Pentateuch - *Leviticus*

**Written Law** – Torah, Pentateuch, Five Books of Moses (*Torah she'bichtav*).

**Yad Chazakah** – see Mishneh Torah (Maimonides)

# INDEX